Dedication

To the memory and aspirations
of Grandmaster Xiong Yanghe
and to all who have carried on
his exemplary blending
of *wen* (文) and *wu* (武)
— the civil with the martial.

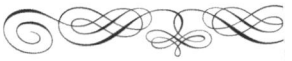

I0616268

Acknowledgments

A special thanks to the following people for graciously contributing to this book in various ways: Masters Chen Deyang, Chen Xiaoyin, Huang Guozhi, Lin Chaolai, Lin Jianhong, and Pan Taichun for providing information and photographs; to my students Debra Rivera and Tan Guangting who appeared in photographs. Above all, a deep bow to Master Xiong Naiqi for kindly providing photographs of his great grandfather Xiong Yanghe, proofreading, and for being so trusting in sharing his family with me. It is an honor.

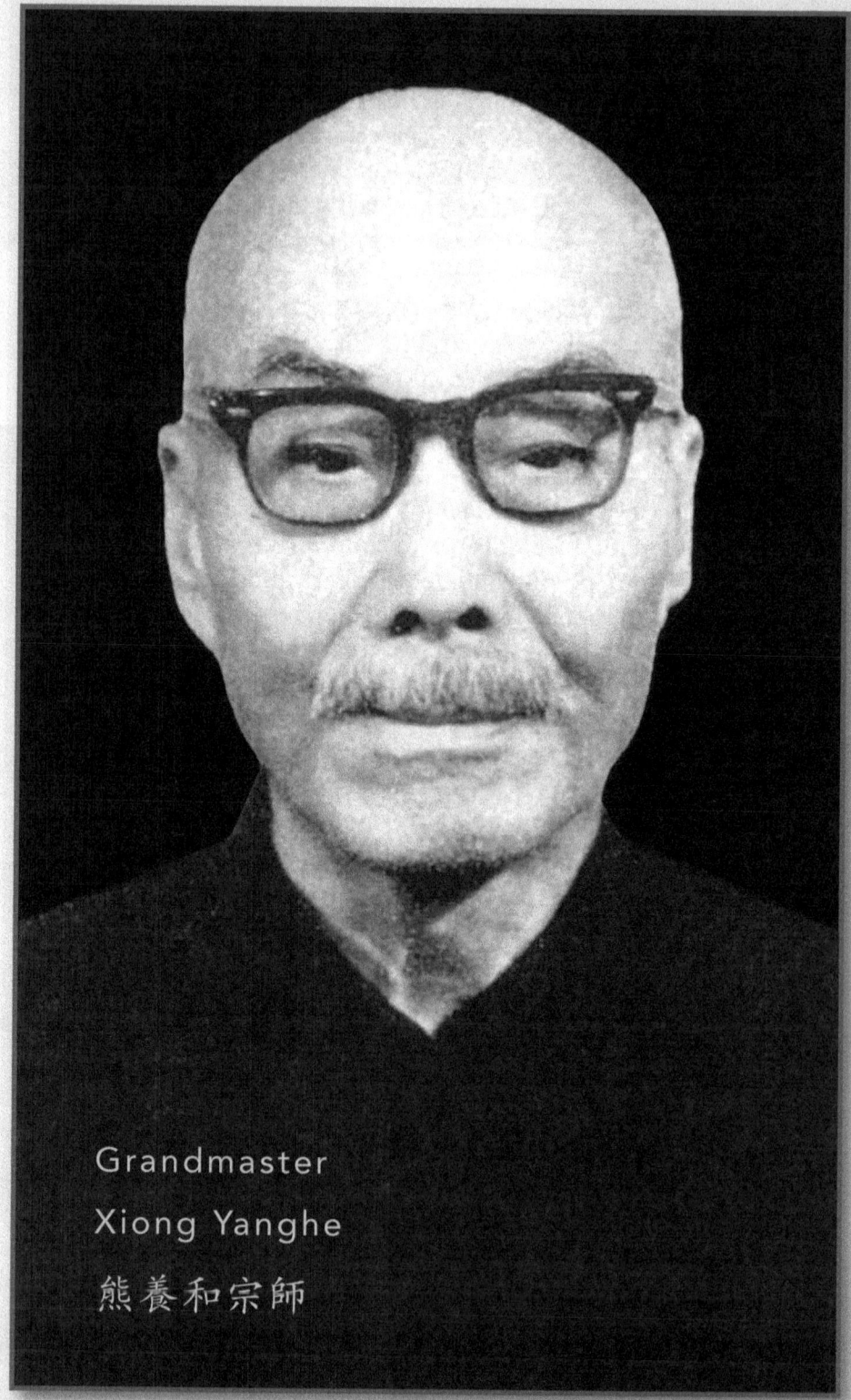

Grandmaster
Xiong Yanghe
熊養和宗師

TABLE OF CONTENTS

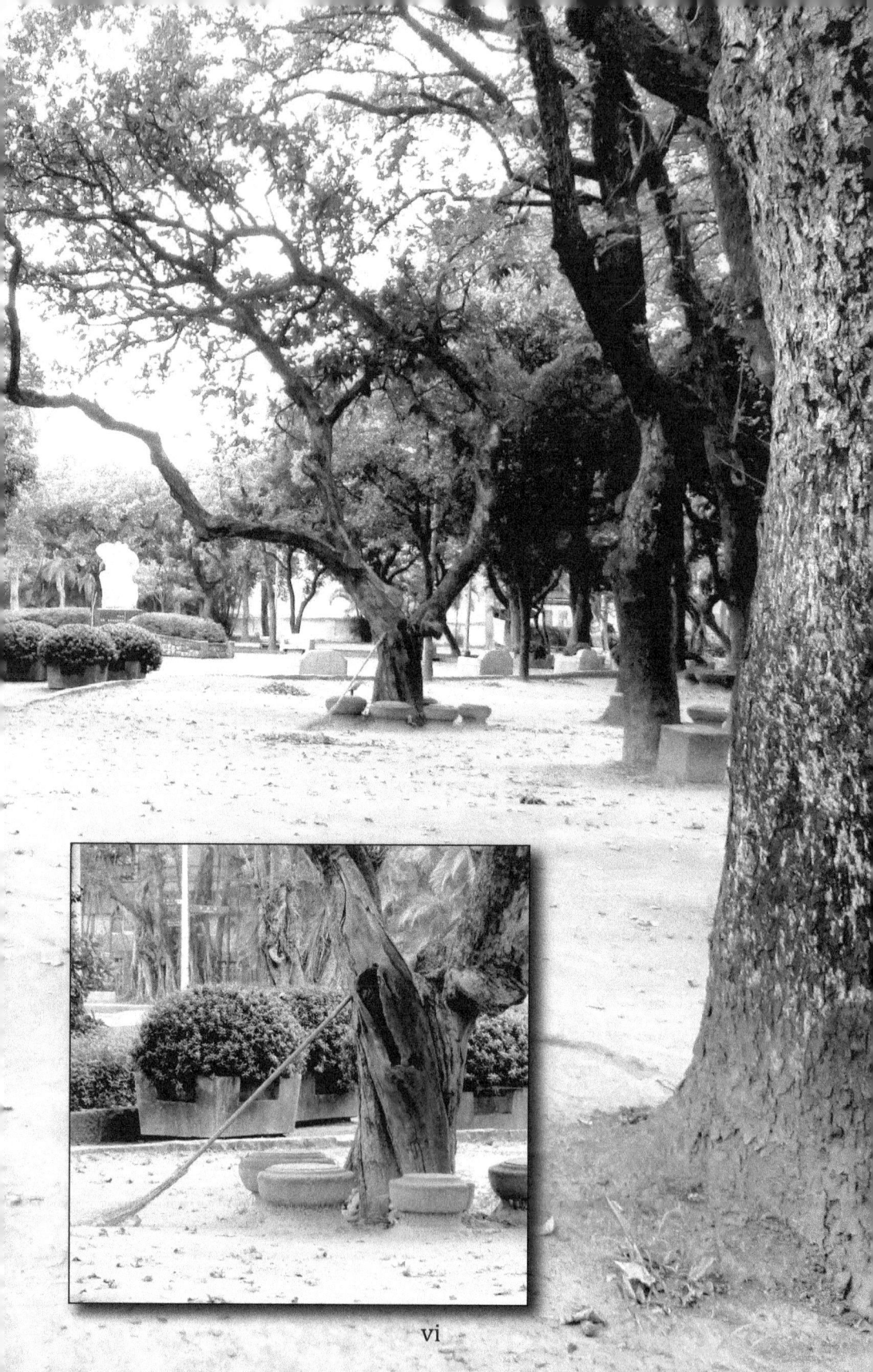

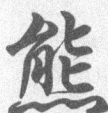
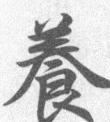
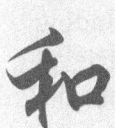
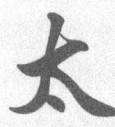
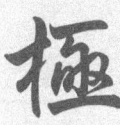
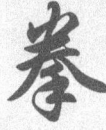

Grandmaster Xiong Yanghe's Taijiquan System

by Michael A. DeMarco, M.A.

▸ long routine ▸ push hands ▸ sanshou
▸ straight sword ▸ broadsword ▸ staff/spear . . .

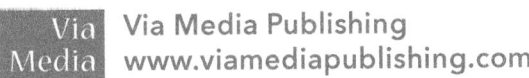
Via Media Publishing
www.viamediapublishing.com

Book and cover design
by Via Media Publishing Company

Cover illustration
Photograph of Xiong Yonghe in single whip posture.
Background texture: File ID 184029145 |
© Angkana Kittayachaweng |Dreamstime.com

ISBN 979-8-218-79352-4

www.viamediapublishing.com

PREFACE

It was a different era back in 1976, when I first flew to Taiwan to study taijiquan. Not many in the English-speaking countries had yet heard of taijiquan's existence. My obsession with martial arts and Chinese culture drew me to the island. I had studied Mandarin in college and my teacher arranged for me to study taiji with Master Yang Qingyu (1915-2002) in Taipei. I had no idea what lay ahead.

We met every weekday morning at New Park, later renamed as 228 Peace Memorial Park. Through the morning twilight streamed people walking to the park—a sort of Shangri-La amid the streets of a quickly modernizing capital city. Mr. Yang arrived and stepped onto the practice ground that nature had provided under the canopy of trees. Worn by years of practice, the ground was only soft dirt, slightly textured with thin lines of hard tree roots. Although Mr. Yang wore no uniform or insignia of rank, people always showed utmost respect for him as a person and as a teacher.

I last saw Master Yang in 1986. He had moved to Puli in central Taiwan and was regularly teaching Buddhist monks. He gave me his own room at his home while he went to the temple to sleep. We spent much time together simply walking, talking, and practicing.

The distance between the USA and Taiwan, plus my limited Mandarin language skill, made it difficult for me to grasp everything teacher Yang had to offer. I knew of his teacher, Xiong Yanghe, and had an idea of Xiong's curriculum. Over the decades, I realized that Xiong's syllabus was much more extensive than originally thought!

In November of 2017, I had participated in the 130th anniversary celebration of Grandmaster Xiong held in Yilan city. Hundreds of Xiong stylists attended, some from overseas. The grandmaster is known everywhere on the island, but little outside of Taiwan because information about him is largely in Chinese and only a few Xiong Style teachers are living and teaching in foreign countries.

For the past fifty years I have gathered as much information as I could about Xiong and his system. It seems a good time to publish some of this material in a book format that could be useful to my students and other English-speakers who have an interest in this specific taiji lineage. May you find this book a good reference and an inspiration for your taijiquan practice.

Previous page: The area where Master Yang Qingyu taught in 1976.

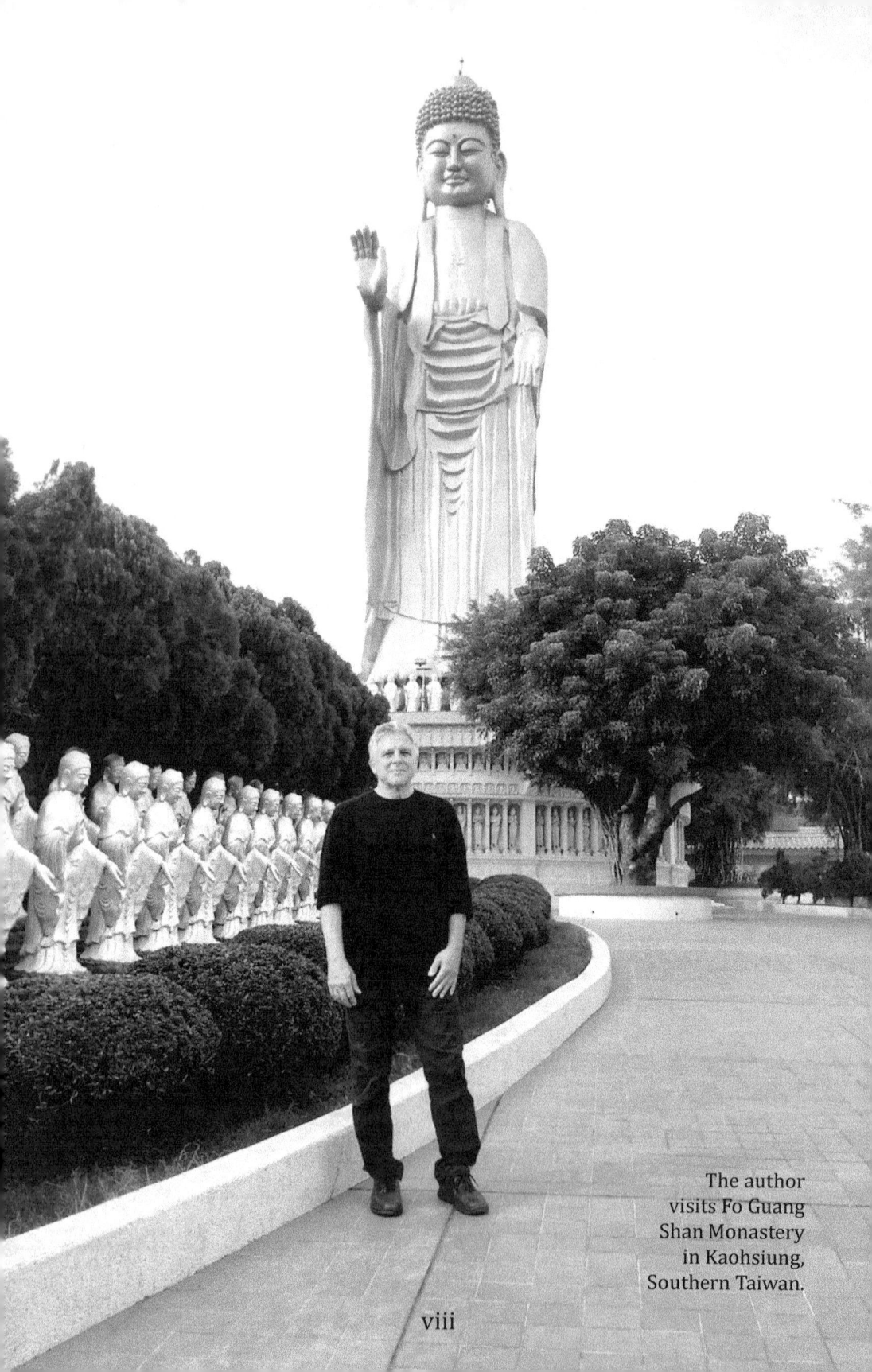

The author
visits Fo Guang
Shan Monastery
in Kaohsiung,
Southern Taiwan.

Taijiquan Enters the Twentieth Century

In the thickly branched tree representing taijiquan's growth over the centuries, some branches are stronger than others, and some hold higher positions than others. This book introduces a relatively rare branch in the Yang Family tradition that is associated with Xiong Yanghe (1889-1981). Before delving into aspects of what is now called the Xiong Style, we must first ask ourselves what we can learn from studying the lives of main lineage representatives. How can their theories and practices of taiji influence our overall understanding of the art? Hopefully such research can offer a better historical perspective while enriching both our understanding and practice of the art.

The following text presents aspects of lineage that play a role in formulating a definition of taijiquan. Following a general overview of the early Yang Family lineage, we will look closely at the two main branches that stem directly from the Yang Style founder, Yang Luchan (1799-1872), his sons and grandsons, who were so influential in the initial growth of taiji in China. Since the focus of this chapter is on Xiong Style, it is necessary to look at Xiong's teachers and these main predecessors who formed the main trunk of the taiji evolutionary tree.

China's socio-political setting during the lives of Yang Luchan and Xiong Yanghe was rife with foreign invasions and civil strife. This difficult period—marred by the decaying decades of the last dynasty (Qing, 1644-1911) and the following decades up to the founding of the People's Republic of China in 1949—presents an overwhelming wealth of information that played into the thoughts and actions of each taiji master mentioned above. Each master has his own story to tell. This chapter gives a brief synopsis of Xiong Yanghe's story.

The Question of Taiji Lineage

Many newcomers are thrilled to begin learning taiji. If they have a decent teacher and a growing interest in the art, they eventually delve deeper into its history, theory, and practice. However, they soon find themselves entangled in a mesh of lineage lines. Who taught whom? What are the differences between the original Chen Family Style and evolving branches? What did the main instructors teach versus the curricula taught by their students in following generations? In the end, what do we really learn from the academic grasp of lineages, names, dates, and a stock of stories which may be true or false?

When we approach taijiquan's history, we are usually given our initial glimpse through our first teacher. This experience introduces one to taiji. Depending on the teacher, the art may be totally focused on its health nurturing aspects suitable for aged retirees in their quest to keep fit. Some teachers focus on it as a fighting art, suitable for bodyguards, military, and police. Others can teach both aspects of the art in varied proportions.

There are other layers to consider in our desire to understand taiji. All teachers have unique qualities in their form and function: movements, stances, fighting techniques, and applied skills. It is easy to see great differences among beginning students in their awkward execution of taiji forms, but even teachers of the same lineage and generation exhibit their own individual flavors, although it may be in the most subtle ways. Of course, it is important to discern the dissimilarity in movements as either a variant application performed according to taiji principles, or an incorrect movement based on faulty understanding of application and performed contrary to the taiji principles.

Often the more we learn about taiji the more confusing it gets! There is an old tale that originated in India that may offer some help in our view of taiji lineages and practice. It is the story of six blind men who were asked to describe the nature of an elephant, with each person feeling the elephant's various body parts, such as its tusk, tail, trunk, leg, ear, or side. Of course, all their conclusions vary because of their different perspectives. The "elephant" they envisioned appeared like a spear, wall, snake, tree, fan or rope. They may endlessly argue over their viewpoints or use them to better understand what an elephant really is in its completeness.

If we really seek to know taiji thoroughly, we need to go beyond relative half-truths to get a broader perspective. A study of the leading standard-bearers of each main lineage is certainly helpful for the broad view. On a more detailed level, we can look closely at the main teachers within one specific lineage. The learning process takes many years, and we eventually see how our concept of taiji continually evolves.

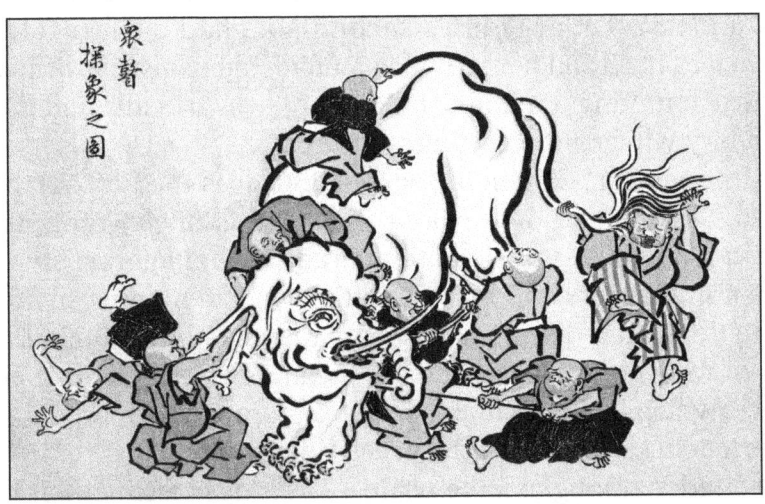

Japanese illustration from Buddhist parable showing blind monks examining an elephant. Dated 1888. Library of Congress. Call # Illus. in H67 [Asian RR]

Early Yang Style Lineage Representatives

Yang Luchan was born in 1799 in Yongnian County, Hebei Province. Although he was a man of humble origins and illiterate, he loved martial arts. He probably studied Shaolin boxing when very young but later was drawn to the Chen Village in Henan Province with the desire to study Chen Family Taijiquan. Although there are a number of stories regarding Luchan's study in Chen Village, the most probable themes are: 1) he worked as a servant and studied Chen Taiji under Chen Changxing (1771-1853) for ten years or so, becoming extraordinarily proficient in the art, 2) he returned to his home village and taught the art to many there, and 3) moved to Beijing where he gained a reputation as "Invincible Yang" and taught the Manchu royal family and bodyguards. Of course, his unique flavor of taiji became known as the Yang Style.

Whether factual or fictional, stories regarding Yang Luchan leave no doubt that he possessed fighting skills of the highest order. What he taught and to whom is another matter. It certainly would be logical for him to follow ancient precedent and teach the higher aspects of the art only to those closest to him.

3

When Yang Luchan died in 1872, two of his sons carried on the family's taiji tradition. Both were naturally gifted, mentally and physically, to receive full transmission of their father's knowledge, and both practiced with dedication under a demanding training regimen. The brothers came to exhibit very different personalities. Yang Banhou (1837-1892), Yang's second son, had a character often described as hard and fierce, which manifested in his love of sparring. The third son, Yang Jianhou (1839-1917), was friendly and gentle, a personality which attracted many students.

Although Yang Shaohou (1862-1930) was the first son of Yang Jianhou, Shaohou studied primarily with his uncle, Yang Banhou. Shaohou followed his uncle in temperament and fighting style. Both were harsh teachers and only a relatively small number of students became dedicated disciples. It seems they used the combative elements of Yang Luchan's methods as the main guideline for their own practice, which included high speed execution of techniques, jumps, and varied kicks, as well as the psychological use of expressions and vocal sound. As Douglas Wile writes: "Writings tracing their origins to Yang [Banhou] are our closest link to Yang [Luchan] and to the richness of the art before it moved into the mainstream of Chinese culture in the twentieth century" (Wile, 1996: 93).

Yang Jianhou's third son was Yang Chengfu (1883-1936). He and his brother Shaohou taught taijiquan at the Beijing Physical Culture Research Institute from 1914 until 1928. They were pioneers in bringing instruction to the public. Chengfu moved to Shanghai in 1928 and taught many. Over the years, Chengfu's style became the most widespread. He eliminated some of the more vigorous techniques from the long routine and taught others to practice at a slow, even tempo. Although he certainly retained the teachings of his father, uncle, and grandfather, Chengfu's public style became popular for its health nurturing benefits.

Lineage Chart Early Yang Family

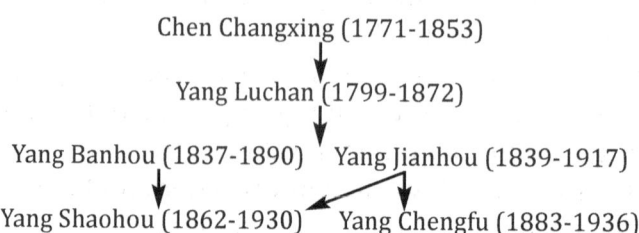

Chen Changxing (1771-1853)

Yang Luchan (1799-1872)

Yang Banhou (1837-1890)   Yang Jianhou (1839-1917)

Yang Shaohou (1862-1930)   Yang Chengfu (1883-1936)

The five Yang family members discussed in the preceding paragraphs lived during a time of drastic change in China. Their lives cover 137 years, from the birth of Yang Luchan in 1799 to the death of Yang Chengfu in 1936. A brief overview of Chinese history during this period will be helpful for understanding the development of taijiquan, as well as other Chinese martial arts that have become popular in the modern era. The realities of those decades influenced the ways the early taiji masters viewed their art, how they taught, and to whom they would transmit their knowledge and skills.

The Effect of Time and Place on Early Yang Style Taiji

What inspired Yang Luchan to study martial arts? Was Chen Family boxing very different from other family styles developed in other villages? Actually, to have a group of villagers with a common surname practicing boxing within their courtyards was not a rare phenomenon in the latter half of the Qing Dynasty (1644-1911). Philip Kuhn (1970) details the growth of local militia, rebels, bandit groups, and secret societies in his excellent work, *Rebellion and Its Enemies in Late Imperial China: Militarization and Social Structure, 1796-1864*. Chen Village is only one example of a village that built up their walls and fighting tradition for protection from attack and theft from outsiders, such as local bandits.

There are "two basic types of militia institutions in Chinese society—those born of state prescription and those born of the needs of natural social units. . .." (Kuhn, 1970: 35). The rise of local defense groups became increasingly important as the Qing government and its military and police structures fragmented under internal and external pressures. Their rise was in direct response to the unstable socio-political climate.

In the 18th century there was a growing domestic discontent throughout China as the population increased to a point where food production could not keep pace. "Population growth inevitably surpassed increased food production, and the standard of living began to decline. Spreading corruption and indolence in government made conditions worse" (Hucker, 1975: 302). Besides an anti-foreign sentiment for the Manchu rulers who conquered China and ruled from 1644 to 1911, the general population felt the government had lost the Mandate of Heaven and was unfit to rule. Popular uprisings became endemic, erupting into major social upheavals such as the rebellion by the White Lotus Society (1793-1804). Even more

5

devastating was the Taiping Rebellion (1851-1864) in which nearly thirty million lost their lives bringing destruction to fifteen provinces (Wakeman, 1977: 156). By the mid-19th century, in some provinces "two-thirds of the population was reported dead or missing" (Wakeman, 1977: 155).

For centuries, China had thought itself to be the most civilized state in the world. However, rebellions, famine, and floods took a great toll on the government and society during the 19th century. China's image of itself gradually changed. It was no longer a country of strength and wealth, and foreign countries took advantage of this frailty. With the intrusion of European traders and missionaries, China soon felt its weakness regarding modern ways of warfare and international business. Over the decades, the Portuguese, Dutch, British, French, Americans, Russians, and Japanese applied more pressure on China as they tried to profit through unequal trade agreements, acquisition of port cities, opium trafficking, and a siphoning off the dwindling reserves of silver. Foreign powers took advantage of a China that had already been weakened from within.

In parallel with a long list of internal rebellions is a list of wars with foreign countries, such as the Opium War (1839-1842), the Anglo-Chinese War (1856-1860), and the Sino-French War (1884-1885). The foreign encroachments were destructive, but their real significance lies in the resulting treaties, which were unequal in that they gave great advantage to the foreign powers at a high cost to the Chinese. The Sino-Japanese War (1884-1895) provided a "profound psychological shock," since it "did more than any other crisis to force the Chinese to evaluate their own strengths and weaknesses" (Wakeman, 1977: 192). Above all, each treaty humiliated the Chinese, and many started to seek solutions to resolve the problems caused by the decades of internal strife and foreign influence.

During the latter half of the 19th century, many political and intellectual leaders were engaged in discussing ways to restore the Qing Imperial system or a new political system through "self-strengthening." It seems most of the attempts either failed or made matters worse. For example, one idea was to use the resentment against imperialist expansion to encourage the Boxer Uprising (1900-1901) against foreign embassies. This was doomed to failure. "Thousands of young men began to practice the stylized exercises of Shaolin and [bagua] boxing—exercises that were supposed to release their [qi] (pneuma) and invest them with strength so awesome that it repelled foreign bullets" (Wakeman, 1977: 217). Even a Chinese military general "simply scoffed at their claims of invulnerability to firearms," and "put 50 Boxers of the Golden Belt Society to the test by lining them up against a wall and shooting them" (Wakeman, 1977: 218). The Boxers' leader was caught and decapitated. Their defeat brought new demands upon the Chinese and resulted in even greater loss of power.

As the Beijing government was losing control of the provinces, there was a corresponding growth of power in local areas, often associated with the provinces themselves. Frederic Wakeman notes that "the provincial governors of the early 1900s, took on more and more of the military and fiscal functions that had once belonged to the central government" (Wakeman, 1977: 232). In nearly half of China's provinces "military men became governors immediately after the [Wuhan Revolution (1911)], or within the following two or three months. Moreover, the troops in the various provinces ... were largely recruited from within the provinces in which they served; their loyalties were strongly provincial and personal, so that provincial military leaders had, in effect, personal armies at their disposal. . .." (Sheridan, 1977: 147).

As private armies developed—some small and some large—warfare increased. "Between 1916 and 1928, the struggle among independent militarists—warlords—tore China into fragments, and the formal political machinery of the republic that had succeeded the monarchy—the parliament, ministries, and so forth—became largely irrelevant to the realities of Chinese political life. At the head of their personal armies, the warlords dominated districts, provinces, and regions, and warred with neighboring generals for additional territory and revenues" (Sheridan, 1977: 20).

War was endemic during this Warlord Period (1916-1928). One writer has "counted more than 400 large and small civil wars in the province of Szechwan alone" (Sheridan, 1977: 88). With such chaos in the land, how would it be possible to reintegrate China under a modern, unified national government? Each warlord faction operated according to his own interests and political ends. One interesting aspect of note is how soldiers were trained. Decorum varied greatly according to group. Some warlords demanded that troops be highly trained while acting with utmost compassion toward the general population. Their honorable code of discipline stressed good treatment toward all and maintaining personal restraint from vices associated with soldiers of poor character. General Feng Yuxiang (1882-1948), for example, "demanded extraordinary physical fitness, and subjected his officers and men to constant and rigorous training to achieve it. . .. He prohibited drinking, gambling, visiting prostitutes, even swearing" (Sheridan, 1977: 74). At the other end of the spectrum were other warlords and their troops who drank alcohol, raped, and robbed at will.

During the dynamic political and military flux of the warlord period, loyalties often shifted between warlords, as well as their officers and troops (Sheridan, 1977: 58). A few factions grew strong while many became weak and disintegrated or were absorbed. Eventually there were two main political parties contending for supremacy: the Nationalists (*Guomintang*) under the leadership of General Chiang Kai-shek (1887-1975), and the Chinese Communist Party, under Mao Zedong (1893-1976). Initially they worked together to end the warlord period and drive out the Japanese, but their differences in political ideology brought on an inevitable civil war (1927-1949).

Chiang Kai-shek, raised during the warlord period, had learned "to revolve all his politics about the concept of force. . .. He had grown up in a time of treachery and violence. . .. There were few standards of human decency his warlord contemporaries did not violate. They obeyed no law but power . . ." (Schurmann and Schell, 1967: 236). Mao also faced this hard reality, and his often-quoted statement is: "Political power grows out of the barrel of a gun." Chiang and Mao fought it out until the Communists emerged victorious in 1949.

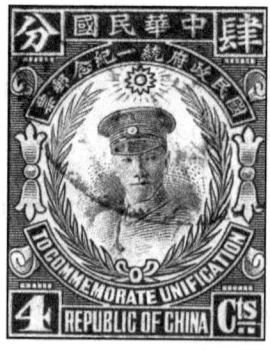

Postage stamp issued by the Republic of China "To Commemorate Unification," bearing the portrait of Generalissimo Chiang Kai-shek.
Courtesy of iStockphoto.com.

A "protracted revolutionary transformation" lasted for more than a century, "but in many ways the critical period was the 37 years, 1912-1949, from the fall of the monarchy and founding of a republic to the establishment of the People's Republic of China by the Communists. During this republican period, disintegration and disorder were at their maximum" (Sheridan, 1977: 4). All the early Yang Style Taijiquan masters lived during this revolutionary transformation, and there are some common factors in their lives that influenced their teaching.

The greatest single factor in taijiquan's development was its association with defense. There were centuries of banditry, small- and large-scale rebellions, and secret society activities throughout China. Particularly, rural areas lacked protection by the national army or police, so martial arts training was utilized for regional and local defense. The Chen Village is only one example of how a family style martial art developed within a walled village, although it is a famous example. It is the site of the original Chen Family Style Taijiquan, which was famed for its superior boxing system. Chen family representatives, such as Chen Changxing (1771-1853) and Chen Gengyun (1799-1872), were employed as elite bodyguards and for cargo transport security personnel; Chen Yenxi (1848-1929) trained the son of the first Republican president Yuan Shikai and was also the family bodyguard for scholar-official Du Youmei in Boai, Henan. Du's son, Du Yuzi (1886-1990) became a disciple of Chen Yenxi.

Fear is a great motivator. People had to protect their food stocks as well as their lives. Many trained hard and often. They also feared a shift in loyalties, so they were cautious about whom they taught. Usually the ties were personal (teaching family or village members) and, under circumstances involving a larger area, ties would be provincial, where common dialect and social customs reinforced some bonding.

The decades of great social change brought changes in relationships. Chen Style moved outside its home village, and others, such as Yang Luchan, came to learn Chen Taiji. Luchan and his son Banhou taught Manchu imperial guards and garrison troops. Some teaching was done privately and some publicaly. "When asked why the [Guangping] students of the Yang family showed both hard and soft techniques in their style, whereas the [Beijing] students showed only soft techniques, [Banhou] replied that the [Beijing] students were mainly wealthy aristocrats, and that, after all, there was a difference between Chinese and Manchus, implying a policy of passive resistance to the alien dynasty by imparting only half of taijiquan transmission" (Wile, 1983: ix).

When Yang Chengfu was born (1883), his grandfather Luchan had already been dead eleven years, and his uncle Banhou died when Chengfu was nine. As a result, Chengfu's training was somewhat different than that of his brother Yang Shaohou. Shaohou and Banhou were noted for their rough boxing. Internationally, Shaohou's style is not as well-known as Yang Chengfu's. The difficulties surrounding his life led him to commit suicide in 1930 (Yun, 2006: 55).

The lives of the Chen Style and early Yang Style Taiji masters reflect their times. The leading figures were highly involved with defense on a local, provincial, and sometimes national level. The need for true, highly effective martial skills was ingrained in the conscious-ness of all facing life and death struggles in their daily lives. Famed martial art teachers, like Yang Luchan, were placed in a quandary between the desire to keep their highest knowledge from "outsiders" and the wish to help close family members and friends. They also had to make a living during difficult times and teaching taiji offered an income.

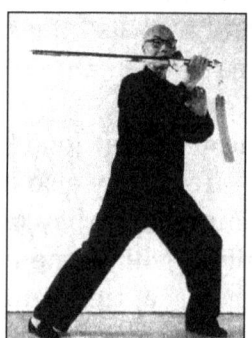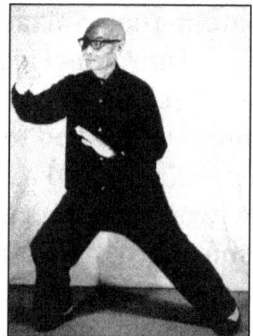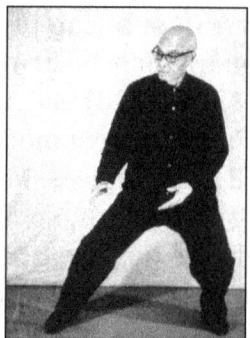

Grandmaster Xiong

There was another motivation for teaching that is often over-looked. It involves the many decades of humiliating treatment at the hands of foreign countries which forced China to give concessions away while losing their own land, wealth, and dignity. The Chinese became known as the "sick man of Asia." That phrase features in the Bruce Lee film *Fist of Fury* (1971), and the Jet Li film *Fearless* (2006). The idea of teaching martial arts for health fit in well with the "self-strengthening" movement in the early 20th century. The country needed to become strong, as did its people.

NOTE References for Chapter 1 follow Chapter 2.

2

Master Xiong Yanghe's Life and Influence

Early on, Yang Luchan and his sons were exhibiting different modes of instruction. They had an array of students: family members, military officials, Manchu guards, other martial art instructors, the affluent and the peasant. Each held the Yang Family tradition and could tailor their instruction according to the student-teacher relationship.

Personalities also played a role in teaching methods as well as in the selection of students. There were polar yin-yang characteristics shown between Yang Banhou (yang) and Yang Jianhou (yin), and in the following generation between Yang Shaohou (yang) and Yang Chengfu (yin)! Shaohou's style was physically and mentally demanding, plus he would not pull punches with his students. Yang Chengfu's style became the most popular because of his more pleasing character and teaching methods. The slower tempo and modifications he made were suitable for a greater number of people, such as the elderly. His teaching had a great impact on national "self-strengthening" by bringing health to thousands.

What is Xiong Yanghe's place in this development? Within the Yang Taiji linage, he took his teachings to Taiwan following the exodus of the Chinese Nationalists to Taiwan in 1949 and became a major influence in the spread of taiji throughout the island. When he passed away in 1981, he and his senior disciples had taught over ten thousand students. His style continues to spread via his disciples, and his unique system is now usually referred to as Xiong Style Taiji. Xiong's story proves interesting for his unique place in taiji as well as his personal life.

Xiong was born on September 29, 1889, in Jiangsu Province, in Funing County. His father, Xiong Weizhen, passed the provincial examination (*juren* military degree) during the late Qing Dynasty. Yanghe studied martial arts first with his father, then his father hired instructors for his young son: at age 12, a Shaolin master named Liu

11

He and his disciple Liu Zhongfang came to teach; at age 15, Master Yin Wanbang for Jiangnan Eight Harmonies Boxing system. These had a martial influence from Gan Fengchi. When Xiong was about 20, "Miraculous Hand" Tang Dianqing (1850-1926) was hired to teach. These teachers provided young Xiong with an excellent foundation in Shaolin boxing and may have given Xiong his first exposure to taijiquan.

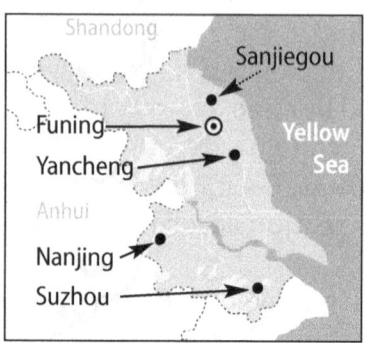

Jiangsu Province is on China's east coast.
Xiong Yanghe was born in Sanjiegou,
which is in present-day Binhai County.

Xiong had hands-on fighting experience as he helped his father maintain township security. He found himself all too often fighting with gangsters. When he was 19 years old, he was the local boxing champion in the "no holds barred" competitions held on raised platforms (*leitai*), as seen in the movie *Fearless*. Because of his powerful kicks, Xiong earned the nickname of "Funing Legs." Such experiences gave him boxing insights, but he was destined to enrich his martial arts by contacts made through his future work.

When Xiong was 23 years old, he began a career in the military, which dealt with security and military operations. At 29, he was Adjunct Director of the Anhui Province government office, and at 35 he went on to a management position in the Funing County garrisons. During this period, Xiong met Yang Style Taijiquan master Hu Pu'an (1878-1947), who associated with many taiji masters of the time. Originally named Yunyu and styled Pu'an, Hu was born in Anhui Province, Jing County. He served as the Department Chief of Jiangsu Province Civil Administration. At the end of the Qing Dynasty in 1911, Hu worked for various publications and helped managed the collection of the Chinese Studies Preservation Society.

As a sinologist well-known for his books and poetry, Hu taught at Shanghai University in the spring of 1924. Afterwards, he became the director of Shanghai General History Museum and the director of Shanghai Literature Committee. Hu was a specialist in philological interpretation and became well known for his work on classics like the *Book of Changes* and the *Book of Poetry*. Hu authored sixty-three works. He was a member of the Nanshe Society, the largest literature and poetry organization in China at that time. Hu also was a co-founder of the Wenmei Society. His expertise was sought after, and he eventually also taught at Chizhi University and National Taiwan University.

While in Shanghai, Hu had an opportunity to meet and study with several high caliber taiji masters. He practiced daily starting at 6:00am for over 18 years, until he became disabled by a stroke and resulting paralysis.[1] Who was Hu's primary taiji teacher? Sources differ, stating he studied with:

1) Chen Weiming (1881-1958) [2]
2) Yang Jianhou (1839-1917) [3]
3) Yang Chengfu (1883-1936) [4]
4) Yang Shaohou (1862-1930) [5]
5) Le Huanzhi (1899-1960) [6]

Most statements regarding Hu Pu'an's teachers simply say that he studied with this person or that one. Furthermore, there are questions about the length of time that Hu studied with his teachers. What could he have learned from them? One reference says "Yang Chengfu and disciple Mr. Hu Pu'an . . . compared notes together, making a thorough study of taijiquan, gaining thorough and penetrating insights into taiji gongfu."[7] To state that Hu was Yang Chengfu's "disciple" is a strong statement. Unfortunately, I have not found solid evidence to substantiate this pronouncement.

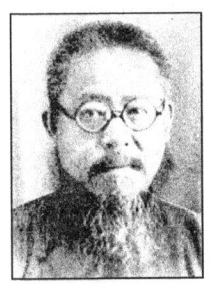

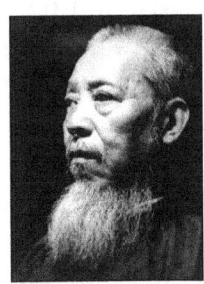

Hu Pu'an (1878-1947).

Left: As editor (1926-1933) of Chizhi Yearbook Press, Chizhi University.

Right: Professor at Shanghai University.

Hu Pu'an probably met all these teachers and may have studied with each to different degrees. But it is interesting to note that he spoke so highly of Le Huanzhi (1899-1960), who was from Gushi County in Henan. Le was a medical doctor and a senior disciple of Dong Yingjie (1898-1961). In his published memoir, Hu wrote that "Le's taijiquan is extremely fine." Hu wrote that—from his own push hands experience with Yang Chengfu, Sun Lutang, Wu Jianquan, and Le Huanzhi—Le proved superior, and his touch was highly effective yet had an undetectable source, "like passing clouds and flowing water," "as not having matter."[8]

Because the sources are obscure, it is difficult to know from whom Hu Pu'an received his taijiquan instruction. Also, the lineage for Xiong has not been evenly defined. There are a few sources, including statements by Xiong's students Liang Dongcai (T.T. Liang) and Zhong Dazhen, that state that Xiong was a disciple of Yang Shaohou.[9] This is also supported by what Xiong taught. Both Xiong and Hu Pu'an had some contact with Yang Shaohou. What we do know for sure is that, in his autobiography (1962), Xiong himself only mentions Hu Pu'an regarding the transmission of the Yang Style Old Frame. This does not negate the possibility that Xiong met other Yang Style Taiji masters or learned their methods via Hu Pu'an.

Xiong may have "studied thoroughly with Hu Pu'an," but he no doubt did have good relations with other taijiquan masters.[10] One source states that Xiong had the chance to meet Yang Jianhou while staying in Beijing for official business. It gave him the opportunity to seek advice about taijiquan, especially regarding the two-person routine call *sanshou* ("dispersing hands"). At this time, Xiong studied wholeheartedly and was able to grasp the deeper mysteries of the art.[11] Yet another source mentions that Yang Jianhou taught in Funing County and Xiong sought his advice for the sanshou practice.[12] Liang Dongcai (aka, T.T. Liang) states that Yang Jianhou taught Xiong sanshou. Liang also maintains that nobody could have possibly learned it from Yang Chengfu, because his father Yang Jianhou died before he could teach it to him (Hayward, 2000: 61).

In his autobiography, Xiong states that had traveled to Hefei, Anhui Province in 1917, where he served as a military commander. He met master Tang Dianqing and others who were taijiquan enthusiasts. Political connections allowed Xiong to meet with Yang family representatives at the governor's office to study *sanshou*. The representatives may have included Yang Shaohou and Tian Zhaolin.

Xiong later amplified his taijiquan studies with Hu Pu'an, who passed on methods from Chen Weiming (including open-hand routines, pushing hands, and weapons).

Since Xiong had to take part in policy discussions falling within the range of his official military duties, he had a great opportunity to meet many people who were highly skilled in a variety of martial traditions. They could compare their studies and benefit by observing the full scope of Chinese martial arts. Over the decades, Xiong received a solid grounding in Northern and Southern Shaolin and taijiquan from his personal teachers and from contact with others through his military career. Here are some highlights from his career:[13]

Age	Position
39	Regimental Commander, Revolutionary Army
40	Jiangsu Province Funing County Public Security Bureau Chief, and concurrent position as Production Brigade Chief
49	Jiangsu Province Funing County Magistrate
52	Security Major General Brigade Commander
53	Security Assistant Commandant
54	Security Major General Commander
58	Major General Group Commander
60	Deputy Commanding Officer, Military Headquarters

In 1949, the Nationalist Party under Chiang Kai-shek retreated to Taiwan and the Communist Party established the People's Republic of China (PRC) on the mainland. Xiong resigned and moved to Taiwan when "nearly 600,000 Nationalist troops and their dependents withdrew from the mainland to Taiwan."[14] It is commonly said that part of this migratory wave included four famed "Big Dogs" of taijiquan: Zheng Manqing (1901-1975), Guo Lianying, Shi Diaomei and Xiong Yanghe.

After settling in Yilan city in 1953, Xiong tirelessly taught taiji. Eventually, Xiong Style practitioners came to number over 10,000. Xiong's most significant contribution to taiji's legacy is the through preservation and transmission of Yang Taijiquan as a fighting art and exercise system, most notably being the two-person practice of sanshou. In addition, his books leave a detailed record of the system.

Even in his twilight years, Xiong was up daily at 4:30 am to start his day, which included his regular taiji classes. In addition to chanting Buddhist scriptures, practicing brush calligraphy, and reading military history, he wrote books, which leave a detailed record of the taiji system for following generations. He was a Buddhist who treated his disciples with a fatherly affection. He died on October 29, 1981, in Yilan Yuan Shan Rongmin Hospital at the age of 94.

Overview of Xiong's Complete Curriculum

On the Neijia Formosa website, David Chesser writes this regarding Xiong's curriculum: "This amount of training makes it the most complete version of taiji practiced on the island. I simply haven't found anything that compares to it."[15]

Xiong's Curriculum

- Yang Family old frame 楊家老架
  Xiong Style Taijiquan (111 Style) 熊氏太極拳111
- taiji basic standing post 太極基本樁
- taiji qigong 太極氣功
- push-hands 推手
- dispersing hands 散手
- taiji straight sword 太極劍
- broadsword 刀
- stick 棍
- staff 桿
- paired straight swords 對劍
- paired broadswords 對刀
- paired sticks 對桿
- paired staves 對棍
- Six Directions Flower Spear 六路花搶
- Spring and Autumn Broadsword 春秋大刀
- double swords 雙劍
- Mizong Boxing 秘宗拳 [迷蹤拳]
- Four Gates Hong Boxing 四門洪拳
- Young Hong Boxing 小洪拳
- Sunlight Palm 曦陽掌等
- and more

The next nine chapters will present Xiong's taijiquan practices including the traditional long routine, push hands, dispersing hands (*sanshou*), staff/spear, broadsword, and the taiji straight sword routine. A following chapter discusses other practices found in the Xiong curriculum today.

Concluding Remarks on Xiong Style Taijiquan

Like the story of the blind men examining an elephant, this chapter can only represent the author's personal findings limited by a relative lack of reference materials, the difficulty in translating Chinese texts accurately, and time available for research. I take responsibility for any shortcomings and welcome any helpful feedback. Hopefully, despite such limitations, the material presented here can broaden the perspective on taijiquan, considering the historical setting where the art was developed by the leading Yang Family lineage representatives.

We have found that there were two major factors influencing early Yang Style development. The first is the nearly incomprehensible violence from the downfall of the Qing Dynasty to the founding of the Peoples' Republic of China, especially during the Republican Period (1911-1949) that soaked the Chinese soil with blood when disorder was at a maximum. It was a time when many sought out superior fighting methods and practiced as if their lives depended upon it. It is no surprise that taijiquan was a desirable system to learn and that it migrated from a small village to be practiced by bodyguards in major cities where military and security personnel were found.

The other major factor influencing taiji's history stems from the exhaustion felt by the country and its population after centuries of rebellions and foreign interventions. Years of struggle, defeat, and humiliation inspired a growing sense of nationalism and an era of "self-strengthening" for the country. One way to cure the "sick man of Asia" was to spread taiji for health: it was found to be highly effective as a form of exercise, no special gear or facility was required, and it was inexpensive when practiced in groups. Millions are healthier because of it.

If we keep in mind the two influences mentioned above while looking at the early Yang Style lineage, a special interrelationship unfolds between taiji and Chinese social history. Between the birth of Yang Luchan and the death of Xiong Yanghe, factions of China's population fought for survival for 150 years before finally emerging as a nation at peace. No doubt Yang Luchan's taiji was a fighting art, but what did it look like? How did he practice? What was the depth of his knowledge?

Most taiji styles today have evolved away from their martial roots. This evolution paralleled the decline of violence in China and the growing social and political stability. At its highest levels, taiji as a fighting art has always been transmitted to a relatively small number of people. Teaching en masse for public health has reached millions. As a result, a vast majority of taiji practitioners know form, but little of function. The reasons one has for learning taiji affects how the form is practiced and looks. We cannot see how Yang Luchan practiced, but the system preserved by Xiong seems to be a good indicator and is valued for preserving a great tradition on Taiwan that was nearly lost during the Communist Cultural Revolution (1966-1976), a social movement that included a crusade to rid China of "old ways of thinking," such as those exhibited in the traditional martial arts.

Xiong Style offers combative elements that were necessary during the extreme chaos found in China during the early Yang Family transmissions of the art. Yang Luchan studied Chen Style and aspects of this are reflected in Xiong Style too: stances are often low and wide, applications are effective, training methods in push-hands and sanshou are practical, and the inclusion of weaponry is encompassing. Even though Xiong's system retains the old Yang flavor, Xiong lived forty years longer than Yang Chengfu and into the post-1949 era. He was motivated to teach for two reasons. He taught close students taiji as a fighting art and as an exercise for health and longevity. Other students were taught basically for "self-strengthening."

This brief overview of Xiong Style helps define and give meaning to the words "taijiquan." Taiji is both an exercise and a fighting art. Its dual nature is inherent in the teachings of true masters. One who has mastered Xiong's system, or the early Yang Family systems, can impart the theory and knowledge applicable in both areas as a combative art and exercise system. The mix is largely determined by the teacher-student relationship and the motives involved. Yang Family Xiong Style Taijiquan gives us a unique opportunity to look back in time when the template of Yang Style was forged. As the system thrives in Taiwan under Xiong's disciples and their own disciples—teachers such as Lin Chaolai, Huang Qinglin, Huang Guozhi, Chen Deyang, Li Guoguang and Lin Qingzhi—we see that the old system has been preserved, while even spreading outside Taiwan to benefit others. It's a taste of "old wine in a new bottle."

18

REFERENCES
Website Sources

1 http://yuehuanzhi.blog.sohu.com
2 www.taiji.net.cn/liu/wlys/200712/6426.shtml;
   http://yuehuanzhi.blog.sohu.com
3 http://blog.udn.com/article/trackback.jsp?uid=wang
   6196192001&aid=107787
4 http://tw.myblog.yahoo.com/q3taichi/article?mid=23&sc=1
5 http://library.taiwanschoolnet.org;
   http://blog.youthwant.com.tw/vadjra/vad-jra/6395839/
6 http://yuehuanzhi.blog.sohu.com;
   www.xici.net/u6819319/d19792891.htm
7 http://tw.myblog.yahoo.com/q3taichi/profile
8 www.xici.net/u6819319/d19792891.htm
9 www.dotaichi.com
10 http://blog.sina.com.tw/lkk_blog/article.php?pbgid
   =36074&entryid=320007
11 http://www.lin-gi.com.tw/discuss/Viewtopic.asp?
   Subject ID=7135&Sign=150
12 http://tw.myblog.yahoo.com/jin_cang/article?mid
   =1003&prev=2170 &next=554& =f&fid=3
13 http://blog.udn.com/wang6196192001/1067085
14 http://taiwanreview.nat.gov.tw/fp.asp?xItem=589&CtNode=128
15 http://chessman71.wordpress.com/2006/05/15/
   yang-shao-hous-taiji/)

People Mentioned

Chen Changxing	陳長興	Shi Diaomei	施調梅
Chen Weiming	陳微明	Sun Lutang	孫祿堂
Chen Yanxi	陳延熙	Tang Dianqing	唐殿卿
Dong Yingjie	董英杰	Wu Jianquan	吳鑑泉
Gan Fengchi	甘鳳池	Xiong Weizhen	熊渭珍
Guo Lianying	郭連英	Xiong Yanghe	熊養和
Hu Pu'an	胡扑(樸)安	Yang Banhou	楊班侯
Le Huanzhi	乐奐之	Yang Chengfu	楊澄甫
Lin Jianhong	林建宏	Yang Jianhou	楊健侯
Lin Shengxuan	林聖軒	Yang Luchan	楊露禪
Liu IIe	劉和	Yang Shaohou	楊少侯
Liu Zhongfang	劉仲仿	Yin Wanbang	殷萬邦

Places

Anhui Province	安徽省	Henan Province	河南省
Chen Village	陳家溝	Jiangsu Province	江蘇省
Funing County	阜寧縣	Jing County	经县
Guangping County	廣平縣	Sanjiegou	三截溝
Gushi County	固始县	Yilan County	宜蘭縣
Hebei Province	河北省	Yongnian County	永年县

References – Chinese

Anonymous (1987). *Mr. Xiong's 100th birthday commemorative special edition.* (n.p.).

Anonymous (1984). *National arts master Xiong Yanghe commemorative collection.* (n.p.).

Lin, Caolai (2007). *Yang family old frame Xiong style taijiquan.* DVD. Yilan, Taiwan: Chin-yu Martial Art Study Association.

Yang, Qingyu (1976). Xiong style taijiquan long form, push-hands, and sword form. Private film collection.

Yang, Qingyu (1988). *Yang Qingyu autobiography.* Self-published.

Yang, Qingyu (n.d.). *A brief biography of Xiong Yanghe.* Self-published.

Xiong, Y.H. (1962). *Xiong Yanghe autobiography.* Self-published.

Xiong, Y.H. (1963). *The taijiquan explained.* Taipei: Taiwan China Book Printing House.

Xiong, Y.H. (1971). *Taiji swordsmanship illustrated.* Yilan, Taiwan: Lu Feng Printing and Publishing House.

Xiong, Y.H. (1975). *The taijiquan explained.* 3rd edition. Taipei: Huge Distribution Planning Company.

References – English

Hucker, C. (1975). *China's imperial past: An introduction to Chinese history and culture.* Stanford, CA: Stanford University Press.

DeMarco, M. (1992). The origin and evolution of taijiquan. *Journal of Asian Martial Arts,* 1(1): 8-25.

Gallagher, P. (2007). *Drawing silk: Masters' secrets for successful tai chi practice.* Charleston, SC: BookSurge.

Hayward, R. (2000). *T'ai-chi ch'uan: Lessons with master T.T. Liang.* St. Paul, MN: Shu-Kuang Press.

Kuhn, P. (1970). *Rebellion and Its Enemies in Late Imperial China: Militarization and Social Structure, 1796-1864.* Cambridge, MA: Harvard University Press.

Kurland, H. (May 1998). "Hsiung Yang-Ho's san shou form." *T'ai chi Ch'uan and Wellness Newsletter*. Downloaded July 16, 2009.

Kurland, H. (2003). "History of a rare t'ai-chi form: San shou." http://www. self-growth.com/articles/Kurland3.html. Downloaded July 16, 2009.

Lu, S. (Yun, Z., Trans.) (2006). *Combat techniques of taiji, xingyi, and bagua*. Berkeley, CA: Blue Snake Books.

Olson, S. (1999). *T'ai chi thirteen sword: A sword master's manual*. Burbank, CA: Multi-Media Books.

Olson, S. (1999). *T'ai chi sensing-hands: A complete guide to t'ai chi t'ui-shou training from original Yang Family records*. Burbank, CA: Multi-Media Books.

Olson, S. (1992). *The teachings of master T.T. Liang: Imagination becomes reality, the complete guide to the 150-posture solo form*. St. Paul, MN: Dragon Door Publications.

Russell, J. (2004). *The tai chi two-person dance: Tai chi with a partner*. Berkeley, CA: North Atlantic Books.

Sheridan, J. (1977). *China in Disintegration: The Republican Era in Chinese history 1912-1949*. New York: The Free Press.

Schurmann, F. and Schell, O. (1967). *Republican China: Nationalism, war, and the rise of Communism 1911-1949*. New York: Vintage Book.

Wakeman, F. (1977). *The fall of imperial China*. New York: The Free Press.

Wile, D. (1996). *T'ai-chi touchstones: Yang family secret transmissions*. Brooklyn, NY: Sweet Chi Press.

Xiong Yanghe Photographs

As part of its goal to maintain cultural records, Taiwan's National Digital Archives Program (see www.ndap.org.tw) has digital photographs of Xiong Yanghe in the collection which can be viewed in thumbnail and large format (view at http:/ digitalarchives.tw).

*Note: Chapters 1 and 2 were previously published in the *Journal of Asian Martial Arts* (2009), Volume 18 Number 3, pp. 18-39.

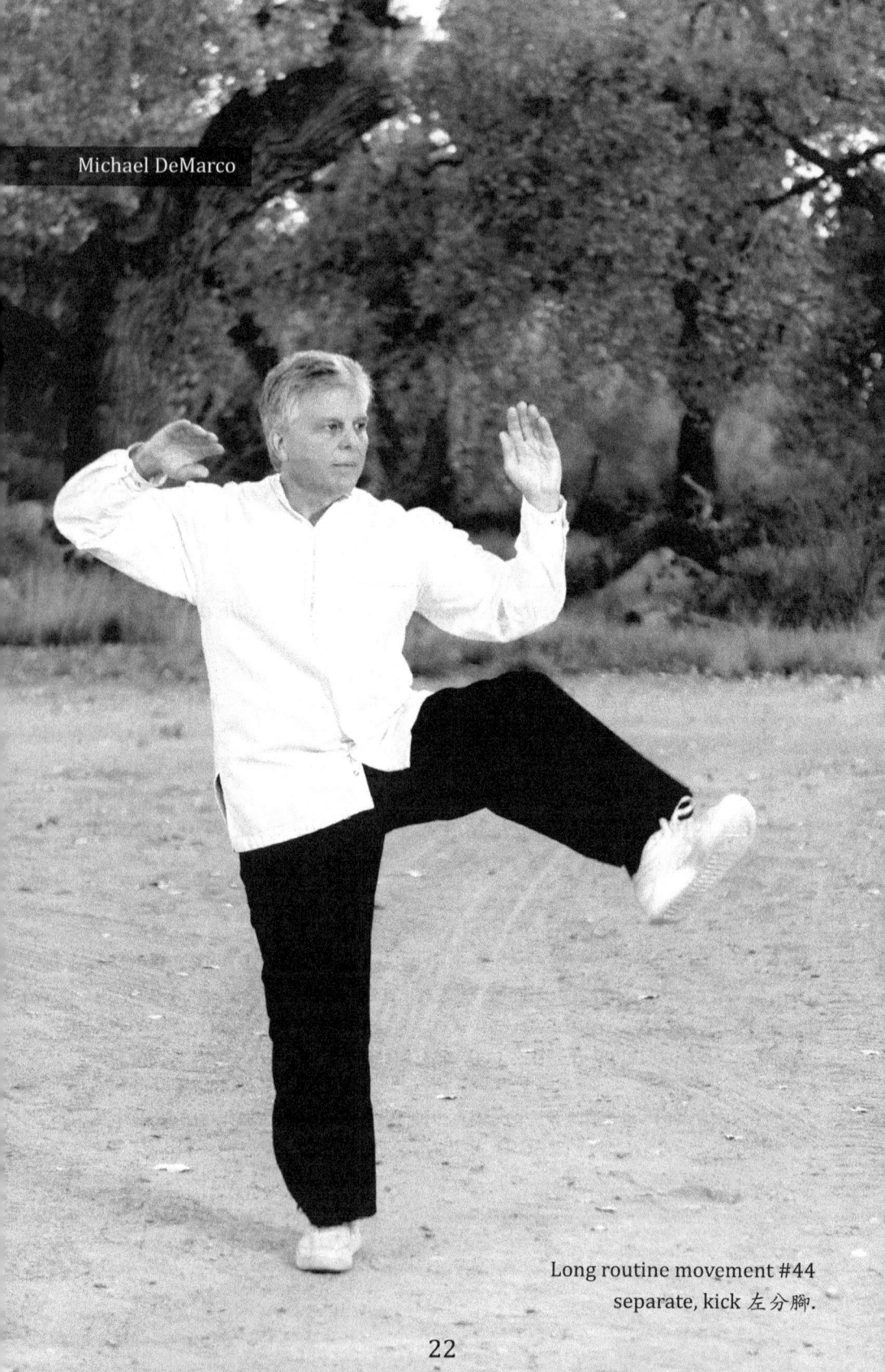

Michael DeMarco

Long routine movement #44
separate, kick 左分脚.

3

Xiong Style Taijiquan Long Routine

The "long routine" is the fundamental taiji practice. It includes over one-hundred martial techniques that are connected by a flow of movement like "pearls on a string." Xiong's taiji long routine is derived from the old traditional Yang Style. Most Yang Style teachers number the movements at 108, mainly because the number is divisible by nine, an auspicious number associated with great success. However, Xiong's numbers the movements at 111 and Xiong style practitioners always refer to it as "Taiji 111."

The long routine is divided into three sections:

- Section One: 23 movements (#1 thru #23)

- Section Two: 38 movements (#24 thru #61)

- Section Three: 50 movements (#62 thru #111)

The long routine preserves techniques which can help students remember the main martial applications in the taijiquan system. Depending on the practice tempo, it can take anywhere from fifteen to thirty minutes to complete the set. The slower tempo is conducive for health aspects noted for the exercise, especially for improved relaxation and balance.

There has been much written about the health benefits from practicing the long routine, so we won't attempt to present them here. Likewise, this book does not focus on instruction or showing the applications of combat techniques. There are high quality books, articles, and videos available for reference.

The following pages present photographs of Grandmaster Xiong as found in the 2018 editions of his three books: *1) Taijiquan Explanations; 2) Illustration of Taiji Sword: Single and Paired Training;* and *3) Taiji Sword Technique Illustrations.*

SECTION ONE • 第一段

1) taijiquan beginning　　　　　　　　　太極拳起勢
2) grasp sparrow's tail (R)　　　　　　　右式攬雀尾
3) ward-off (L)　　　　　　　　　　　　左掤式
4) grasp sparrow's tail (L)　　　　　　　左式攬雀尾
5) ward-off (R)　　　　　　　　　　　　右掤式
6) roll back (L)　　　　　　　　　　　　左将式
7) press (R)　　　　　　　　　　　　　右擠式
8) two-hand push　　　　　　　　　　　右按式
9) single whip　　　　　　　　　　　　左單鞭
10) rising hands　　　　　　　　　　　提手上勢
11) white crane spreads wings　　　　　白鶴掠翅
12) brush knee, twist step (L)　　　　　左摟膝拗步
13) play lute　　　　　　　　　　　　　手揮琵琶
14) brush knee, twist step (L)　　　　　左摟膝拗步
15) brush knee, twist step (R)　　　　　右摟膝拗步
16) brush knee, twist step (L)　　　　　左摟膝拗步
17) play lute　　　　　　　　　　　　　手揮琵琶
18) embrace moon　　　　　　　　　　懷中抱月
19) turn and strike　　　　　　　　　　撇身捶
20) advance, deflect, punch　　　　　　上步搬攔捶
21) withdraw and push　　　　　　　　如封似閉
22) embrace tiger, return to mountain　轉身抱虎歸山
23) cross hands　　　　　　　　　　　十字手

SECTION TWO • 第二段

24) turn and strike　　　　　　　　　　轉身撇身捶
25) ward-off, roll back, press, push　　掤将擠按
26) turn left, sidelong single-whip　　左轉斜單鞭
27) fist under elbow　　　　　　　　　肘底捶
28) repulse monkey (R)　　　　　　　　右式倒攆猴
29) repulse monkey (L), repeat 28-29　左式倒攆猴
30) diagonal flying posture　　　　　　斜飛勢
31) rising hands, step forward　　　　　提手上勢
32) white crane spreads wings　　　　　白鶴掠翅
33) brush knee, twist step (L)　　　　　左摟膝拗步

34) sea bottom probe	海底針
35) fan through the back	扇通背
36) turn and strike	轉身撇身捶
37) advance, deflect and punch	進步搬攔捶
38) advance, ward-off, roll back, press, push	上步掤挒擠按
39) single-whip	單鞭
40) cloud hands (3x)	雲手
41) single-whip	單鞭
42) pat a high horse	高探馬
43) separate kick (R)	右分腳
44) separate kick (L)	左分腳
45) turn, heel kick	轉身蹬腳
46) brush knee (L and R), twist step	左右摟膝拗步
47) advance, planting strike	進步栽捶
48) white snake spits	白蛇吐信
49) advance, evade, punch	進步搬攔捶
50) kick (R)	右踢腳
51) step back, strike tiger (L)	倒插步左打虎
52) strike tiger (R)	右打虎
53) dredge ocean for moon, kick (R)	海底撈月右蹬腳
54) double gusts penetrate ears	雙風貫耳
55) kick (L)	左蹬腳
56) spin around, kick (R)	轉身右蹬腳
57) turn and strike	撇身捶
58) advance, deflect and punch	進步搬攔捶
59) apparent closing	如封似閉
60) embrace tiger, return to mountain	抱虎歸山
61) cross hands	十字手

SECTION THREE • 第三段

62) turn and strike	轉身撇身捶
63) ward-off, roll back, press, push	掤挒擠按
64) single whip	橫單鞭
65) part wild horse's mane (R)	右野馬分鬃
66) part wild horse's mane (L)	左野馬分鬃
67) part wild horse's mane (R)	右野馬分鬃
68) grasp sparrow's tail (L)	左攬雀尾

69) ward-off, roll back, press, push	上步掤捋擠按
70) single whip	單鞭
71) jade lady threads shuttle (1)	玉女穿梭一
72) jade lady threads shuttle (2)	玉女穿梭二
73) jade lady threads shuttle (3)	玉女穿梭三
74) jade lady threads shuttle (4)	玉女穿梭四
75) grasp sparrow's tail (L)	左攬雀尾
76) advance, ward-off, roll back, press, push	上步掤捋擠按
77) single whip	單鞭
78) cloud-hands (3x), cross hands	十字手
79) single whip	單鞭
80) snake creeps down	蛇身下勢
81) golden rooster stands on one leg (R)	右金雞獨立
82) golden rooster stands on one leg (L)	左金雞獨立
83) repulse monkey (L)	倒攆猴
84) diagonal flying posture	斜飛勢
85) rising hands	提手上勢
86) white crane spreads wings	白鶴掠翅
87) brush knee, twist step (L)	摟膝拗步
88) sea bottom probe	海底針
89) fan through the back	扇通背
90) turn and strike	轉身撇身捶
91) advance, deflect and punch	進步搬攔捶
92) advance, ward-off, roll back, press, push	上步掤捋擠按
93) single whip	單鞭
94) cloud-hands (3x)	雲手（大）
95) single whip	單鞭
96) pat a high horse	高探馬
97) cross hands	十字手
98) turn, cross hands, kick	轉身十字腿
99) brush knee, point strike	摟膝指襠捶
100) advance, ward-off, roll back, press, push	上步掤捋擠按
101) single whip	單鞭
102) snake creeps down	蛇身下勢
103) advance to seven stars	上步七星
104) yielding step, ride tiger	退步跨虎
105) turn, lotus sweep	轉身擺蓮

106) bend bow, shoot tiger   彎弓射虎
107) turn and strike   撇身捶
108) advance, deflect and punch   上步搬攔捶
109) apparent closing   如封似閉
110) embrace tiger, return to mountain   轉身抱虎歸山
111) cross hands closing   十字手

Grandmaster Xiong • Section 1 Movements

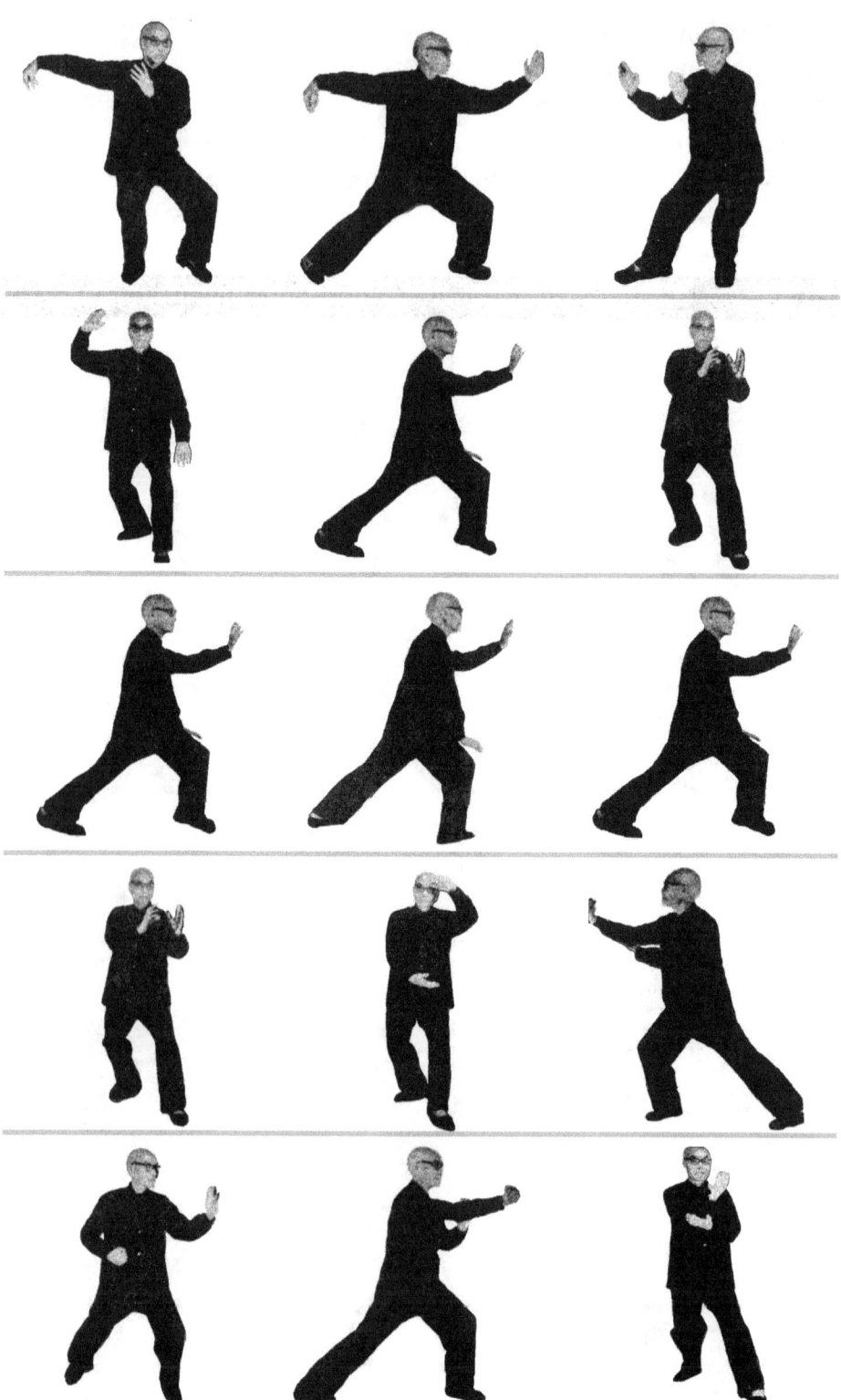

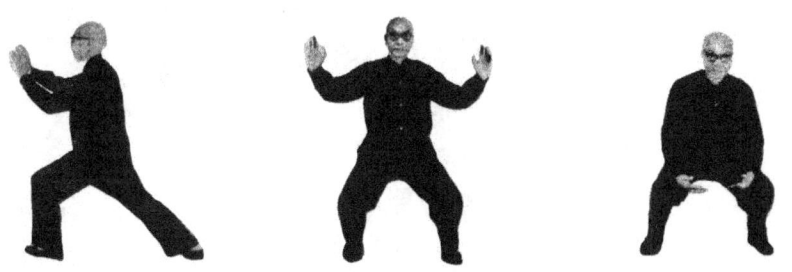

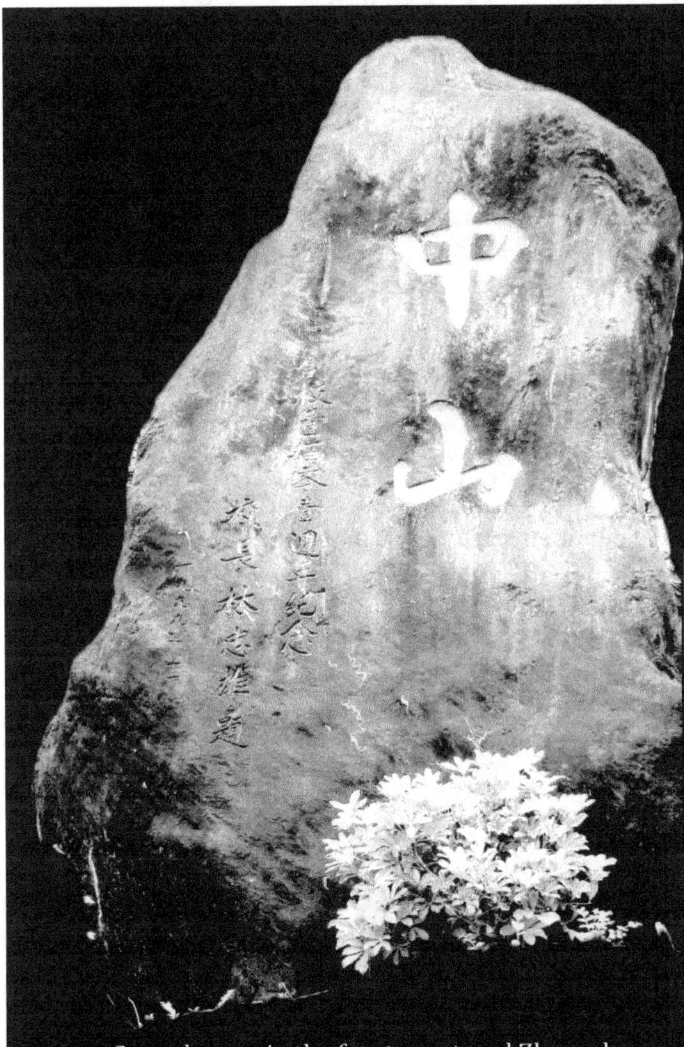

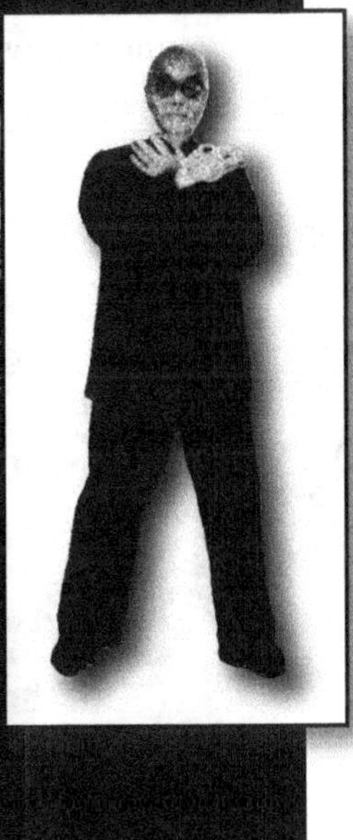

Carved stone in the front courtyard Zhongshan
Elementary School in Yilan. Grandmaster
Xiong taught in this location for many years.

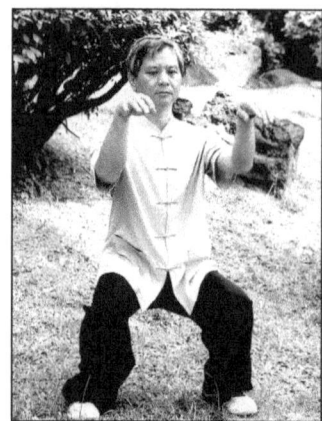
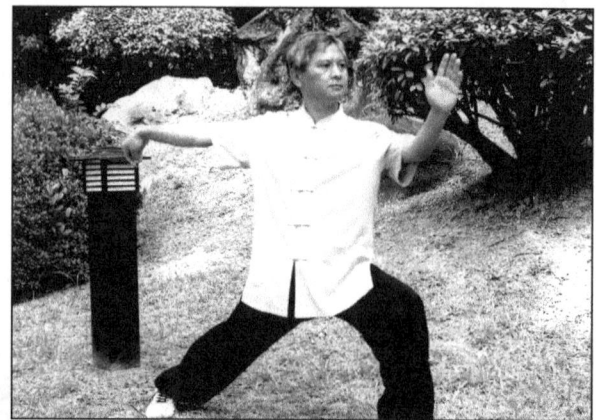
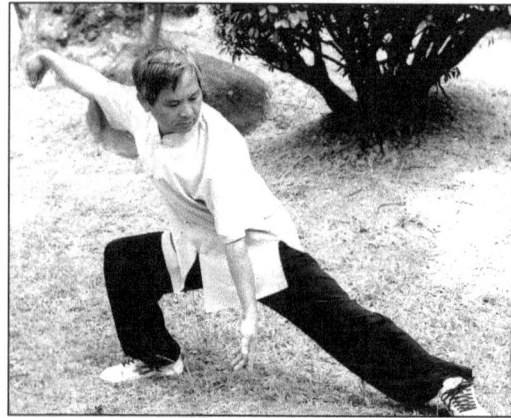
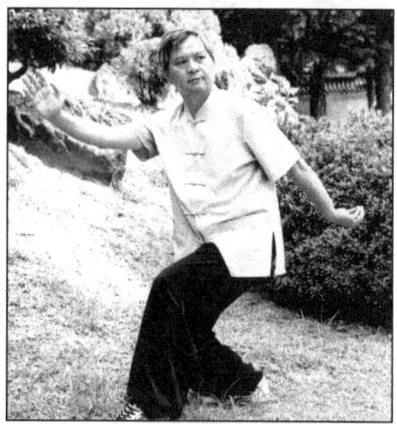

Above, second generation Master Lin Jianhong at solo practice,
and below, a group of his students being led by Ms. Ye Jinxiu.

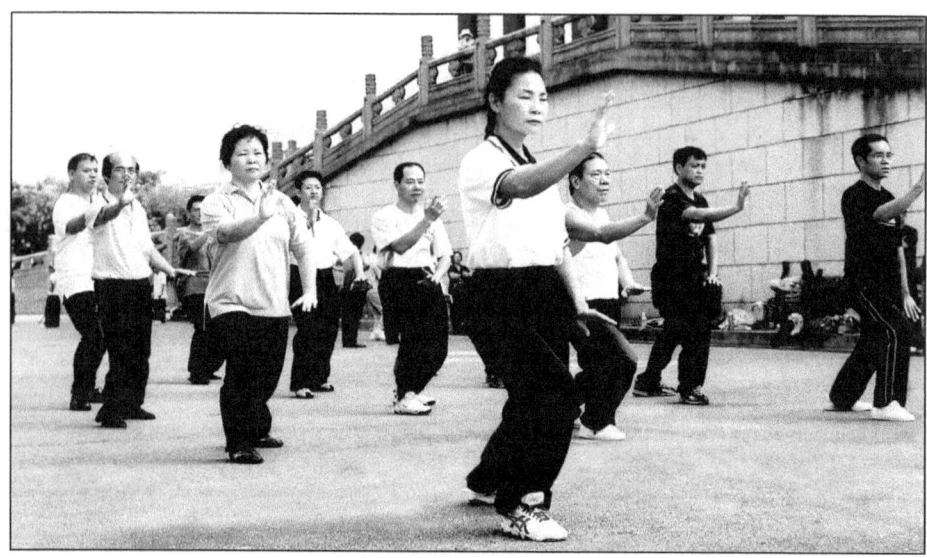

◀ 4 ▶

Push-Hand Methods

The long routine teaches the practitioner how to move properly. How does the direction of the waist relate to the hands and feet? How to step forward, backward, or in circular patters? Hopefully with awareness of each movement, the body and mind can flow in harmony in the execution of each movement in the routine.

There is a progression in taiji pedagogy with the original aim for taiji to be a truly effective martial art. Following the solo form, two-person practices are necessary. Even if the goal is to maintain good health, push hands can be a beneficial practice that is also highly enjoyable.

Push-hands training involves a variety of short, organized patterns between two people utilizing movements contained in the long routine, mainly the basic techniques of ward-off, roll-back, press, and push (*peng, lu, ji, an*) and grab, wring, elbow and shoulder strike (*cai, lie, zhou, kao*). These allow the practitioner to understand the different martial functions and apply them in each cardinal direction.

The pushing methods start without stepping. The practitioners face each other with one arm extended, with their forearms slightly touching. Techniques are performed to sense pressures and tensions with the goal to keep oneself balanced and relaxed.

After four one-hand routines are learned to satisfaction, there are nine two-handed routines with the feet remaining fixed. Then follow four methods that include moving steps, and an additional three versions of *dalu* (large rollback). All these methods teach footwork and develop the ability to move smoothly in the four corner directions.

The final stage in push hands is free form, when partners improvise spontaneously. This requires a high sensitivity to maintain balance and relation while causing the opponent to become tense and attempting to off-balance them. It is a way of mutual learning.

31

Fixed-step single-hand pushing methods   定步單手推法
1) press, neutralize, and push   單手按化推法
2) vertical circle push   單手立圓推法
3) vertical circle up-down push   單手立圓上下推法
4) folding, piercing point, push   單手摺疊穿點推法

Fixed-step two-hand pushing methods   定步雙手推法
1) horizontal circle, stick and push   雙手平圓沾黏推法
2) press, roll back, push   雙手按将推法
3) mutual roll back, push   雙手互将推法
4) roll back, squeeze, horizontal squeeze, push   雙手将擠橫擠推法
5) folding push   雙手摺疊推法
6) squeeze, roll back, neutralize, push   擠将鬆化推法
7) ward-off, roll back, press, push, four directions   掤将擠按四手推法
8) (l, r) ward-off, roll back, push, neutralize, push   左右掤将按化推法
9) press-squeeze, neutralize, roll back, push   按擠化将推法

Push-hands with moving steps   活步推手
1) rotating advance-retreat push   雙手旋轉進退推法
2) closing step, advance-retreat push   雙手合步進退推法
3) following-step spiral push   順步旋繞推法
4) closing step, spiral push   合步旋繞推法

Dalu (large rollback)   大将
1) fixed step, large roll back, press   固定大将之按手推法
2) fixed step, large roll back, fan hands   固定大将之閃手推法
3) free step, large roll back   不固定大将之推法

Free form push-hands   不固定推手

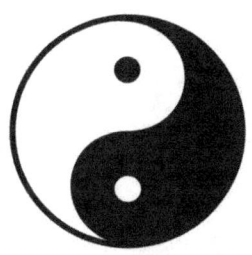

Push-hands: the interaction of yin and yang.

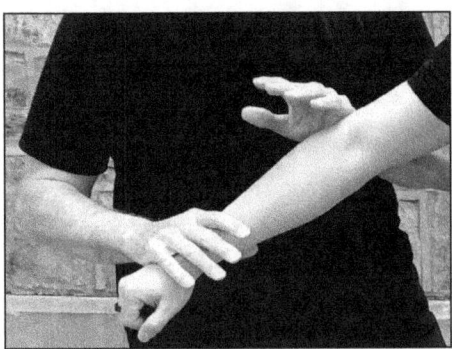

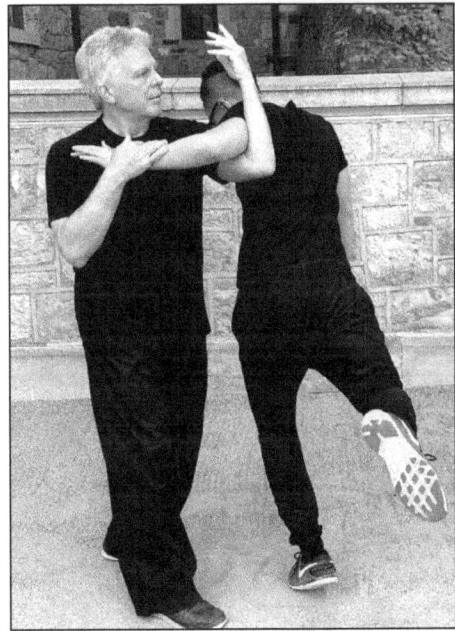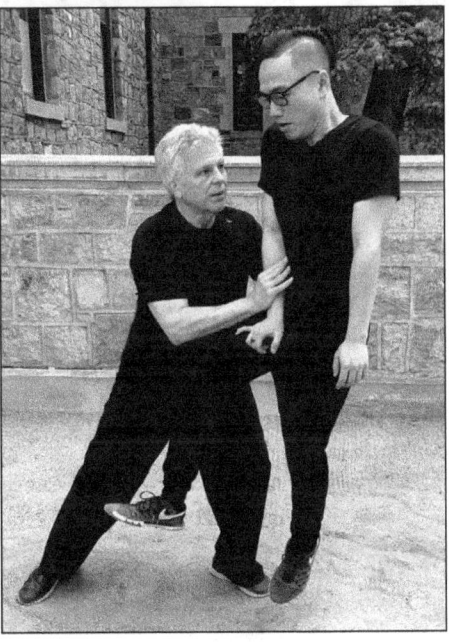

The author and his student, Tan Guangting, practicing free-form push hands, sensing and spontaniously utilizing the applications from the push hand routines and long routine. *Photography by Gail Springer.*

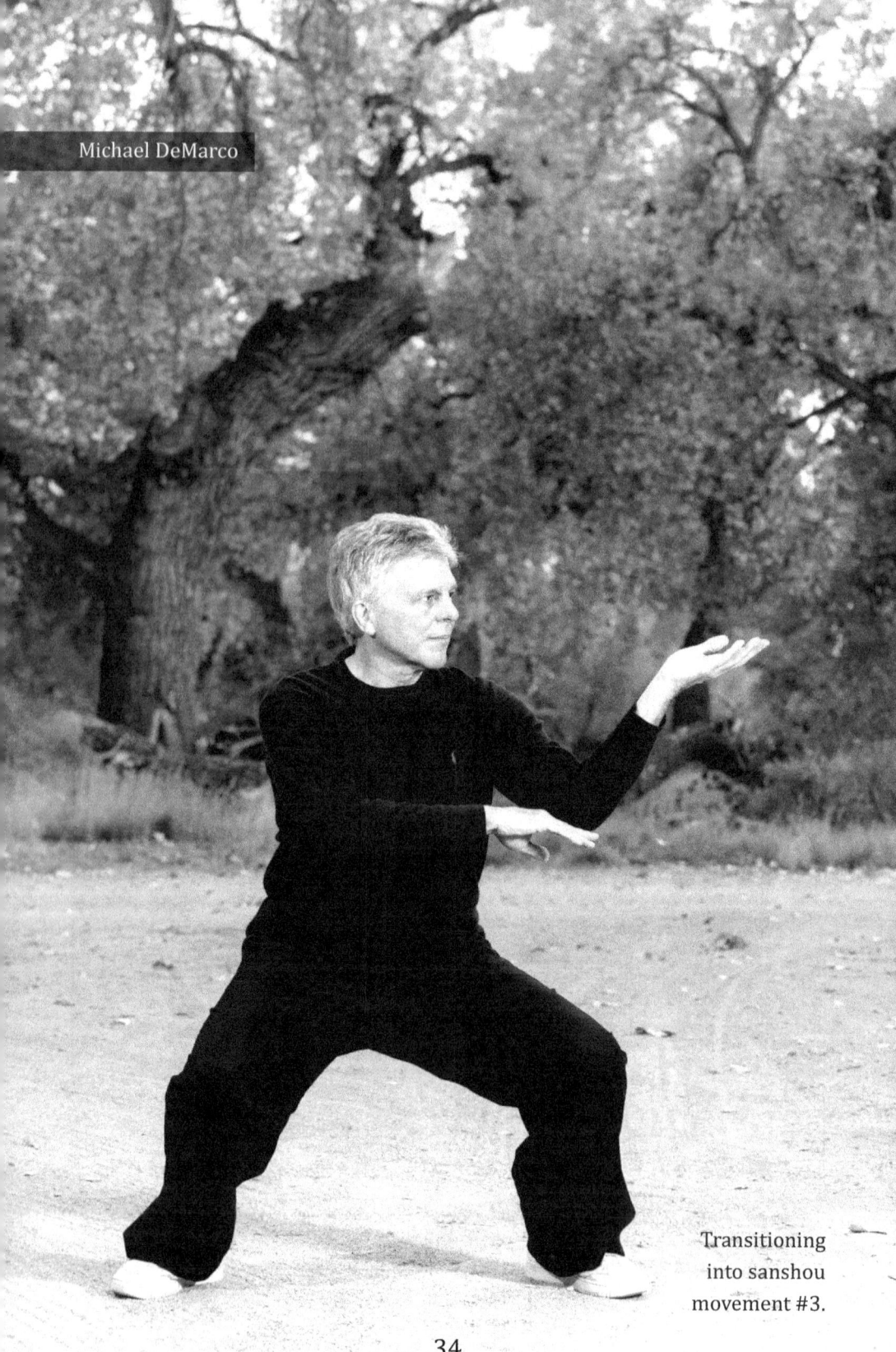

Michael DeMarco

Transitioning into sanshou movement #3.

5

Dispersing Hands Routine (solo/paired)

Sanshou or "dispersing hands" is another step on the progression of taijiquan learning. It takes the practitioner beyond the solo form and push hands methods. Sides A and B can be practiced as solo routines. As a paired routine, it includes the sensitivity of push hands with more applications and extensive footwork taking the practitioner closer to actual combat situations.

The routine starts with opponents facing each other and one side attacks and the other defends. Upon the first touch, the series of attacking and defending alternates between the two partners. Each movement teaches not only how to attack, but also how to defend.

Working with different partners gives one the experience of adapting to different heights, weights and varied direction of movement. Speed varies too. While adapting to each instance (punches, kicks, locks, pushes, pulls, etc.), the practitioner should maintain the primary characteristics of the art—mainly relaxation, balance, and the ability to flow according to the everchanging circumstances. Of course, sanshou is not practiced as slowly as the long routine but is usually performed at medium tempo as in push hands or faster.

Master Xiong most likely had some instruction from Yang Jianhou but had opportunities to practice with other masters as well. The martial aspect is pronounced in sanshou where the fighting applications are clearly seen. What many fail to see and therefore fail to employ are the main principles of taiji as a fighting art. Most will rely on common "hard methods" of blocking and striking, using muscle instead of the potential power of unified body movement stemming from relaxation and speed.

In former times, sanshou was seriously practiced to develop the advanced skills associated with taijiquan for combat usage. Today, many practitioners lack the practical experience for doing this. They practice mainly for the enjoy of movement and for healthful flexibility sanshou provides as an exercise.

1) step forward, punch   上步捶
2) step forward, block, punch   上步攔捶
3) step forward, shoulder strike   上步靠
4) strike with left elbow   打左肘
5) left splitting body punch   左劈身捶
6) retreat step, left strike tiger   撤步左打虎
7) lift hands   提手上式
8) splitting body punch   劈身捶
9) right horizontal split hand   右橫捌手
10) low posture, right hit the tiger   下式右打虎
11) step forward, left shoulder strike   上步左靠
12) double separate kick   雙分蹬腳
13) step forward, right pluck, split   上步右採捌
14) left ward off, right split, strike   左棚右劈身捶
15) step forward, left shoulder strike   上步左靠
16) turn and roll back   轉身按将势
17) step forward, two-hand push   進步雙按
18) single push, right arm   单推右臂
19) follow and push   順势按
20) neutralize and push   化推
21) entering step, pluck and split   進步採捌
22) right strike the tiger   右打虎
23) step forward, left press   上步左擠
24) change step, double open, right shoulder strike 換步雙分右靠
25) right elbow strike   打右肘
26) step back and neutralize   退步化
27) retreat, turn, advance, shoulder strike   後退轉身上步靠
28) turn, change step, right kick   轉身換步右分脚
29) turn, change step, left kick   轉身換步左分脚
30) change hand, right shoulder strike   換手右靠
31) step forward, left grasp sparrow's tail   上步左攬雀尾
32) step forward, right grasp sparrow's tail   上步右攬雀尾
33) right open, left ward-off, right split, strike   右開左棚右劈身捶
34) step forward, pat high horse, left heel kick   上步高探馬左蹬脚
35) turn, lotus kick   轉身摆莲
36) snake moves downward   蛇身下势

37) left strike the tiger	左打虎
38) repulse the monkey (1)	倒撵猴一
39) repulse the monkey (2)	倒撵猴二
40) repulse the monkey (3)	倒撵猴三
41) needle at sea bottom	海底针
42) play pipa	手揮琵琶
43) turn, right single whip	轉身右单鞭
44) step forward, cross arms	上步十字手
45) turn, step back, roll back	轉身退步捋
46) step forward, turn, ride the tiger	上步轉身跨虎

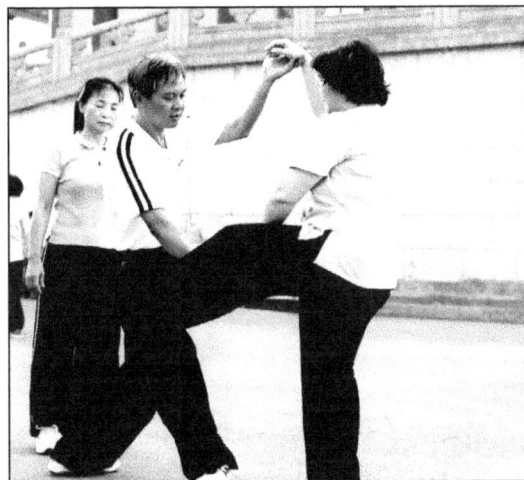
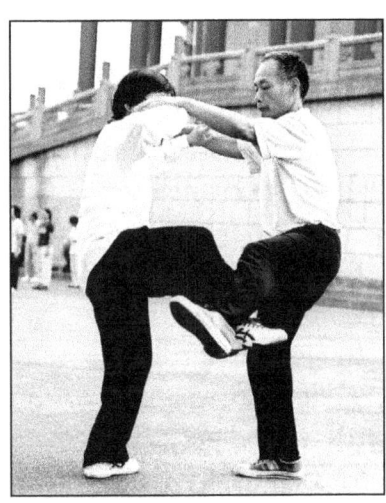
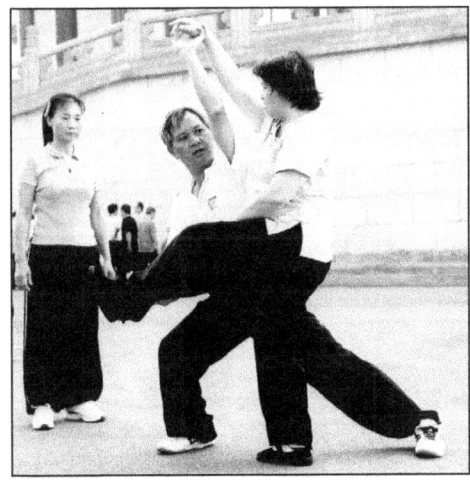
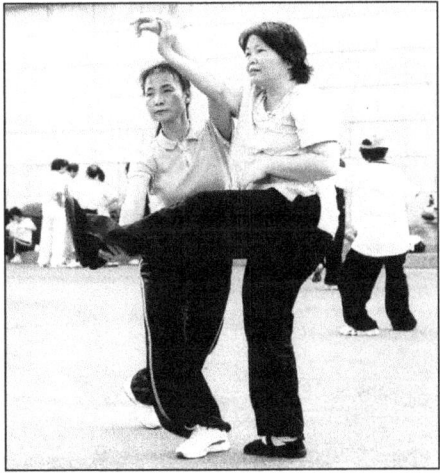

Master Lin Jianhong teaching subtleties of sanshou to his students
at the National Chiang Kai-shek Memorial Park in Taipei, Taiwan.

1) lift hands (beginning posture)   提手上势

2) parry and punch   搬捶

3) strike the tiger right   右打虎

4) push right   右推

5) step back, right shoulder strike   换步右靠

6) right splitting strike   右劈身捶

7) turn and push   轉身按

8) open parry and punch   開勢搬捶

9) part the horse's mane left   换步左野馬分鬃

10) turn, step back, roll back   轉身撤步捋

11) turn right and press   向右轉身按

12) punch to the groin   指襠捶

13) change step, shuttle right   换步右穿梭

14) white crane spreads its wings, left heel kick   白鶴亮翅左蹬脚

15) step back, strike with left arm   撤步撅左臂

16) double gusts strike opponent's ears   雙風貫耳

17) low parry, strike   下勢搬捶

18) right arm roll   右搓臂

19) neutralize, strike with palm strike   化打右掌

20) neutralize, strike with right elbow   化打右肘

21) step back, strike with left arm   换步撅右臂

22) turn, step back, roll back   轉身撤步捋

23) press   回挤

24) step back, turn, left shoulder stroke   换步转身左靠

25) golden rooster stands on one leg   转身金鸡独立

26) two-handed deflection, step forward, left heel   双分上步左蹬脚

27) step back, strike with left arm   退步撅左臂

28) brush knee (R)   双分右摟膝

29) brush knee (L)   双分左摟膝

30) shoulder stroke   回靠

31) cloud hands (R)   右云手

32) cloud hands (L)   左云手

33) strike splitting punch   侧身撅身捶

34) white crane spreads wings, right leg sweep   白鶴亮翅右套腿

35) diagonal flying (L)   左斜飞式

36) diagonal flying (R)   右斜飞式

37) turn, splitting punch 转身撇身捶

38) step forward, left fan hands 上步左搌

39) step forward, right fan hands 上步右搌

40) step forward to the seven stars 上步七星

41) fan through the back 扇通背

42) draw the bow, shoot the tiger 弯弓射虎

43) punch under elbow 肘底捶

44) embrace tiger, return to mountain 抱虎归山

45) step forward, turn, roll back 上步转身捋

46) turn, step back, strike the tiger 轉身退步跨虎

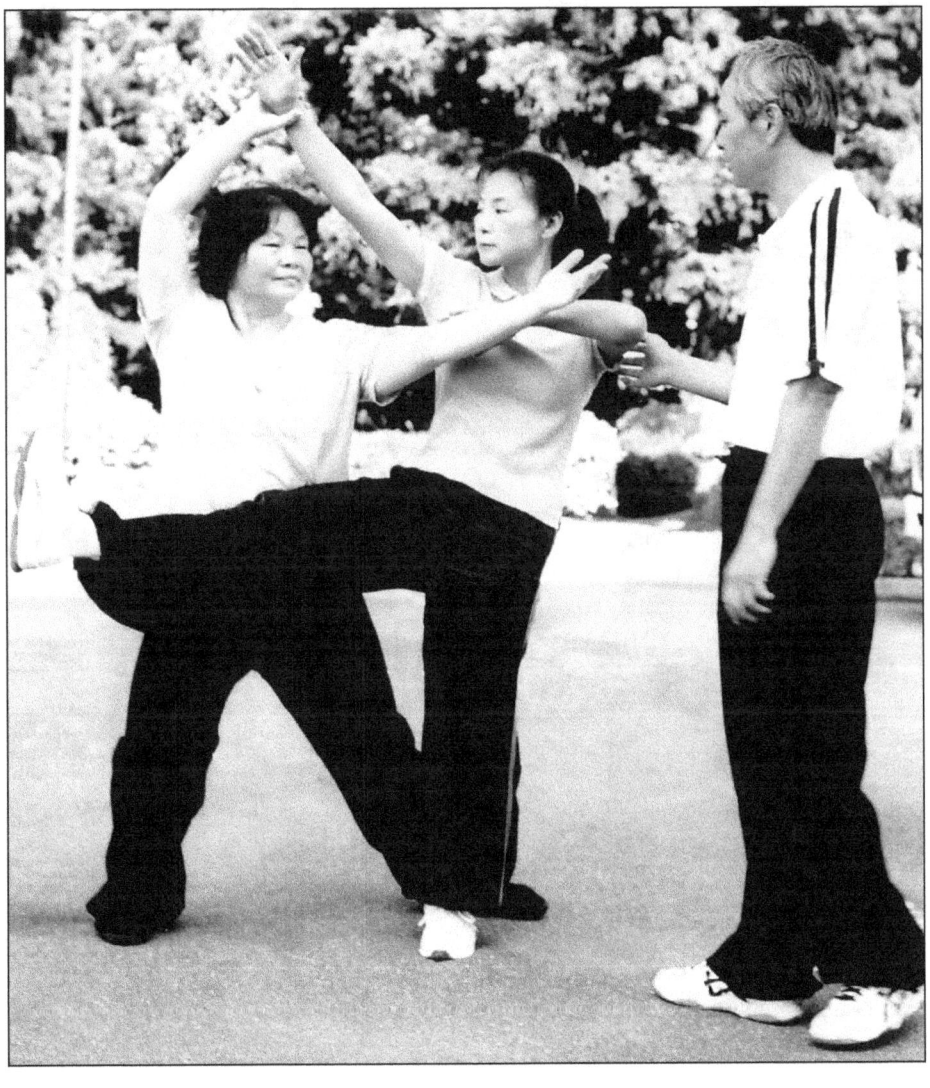

Sanshou

Historic photographs from Grandmaster Xiong's book, *An Interpretation of Taijiquan* (1963 edition). He was about 74 years old when these photographs were made. His student Lin Lianfu (林連富) is his partner.

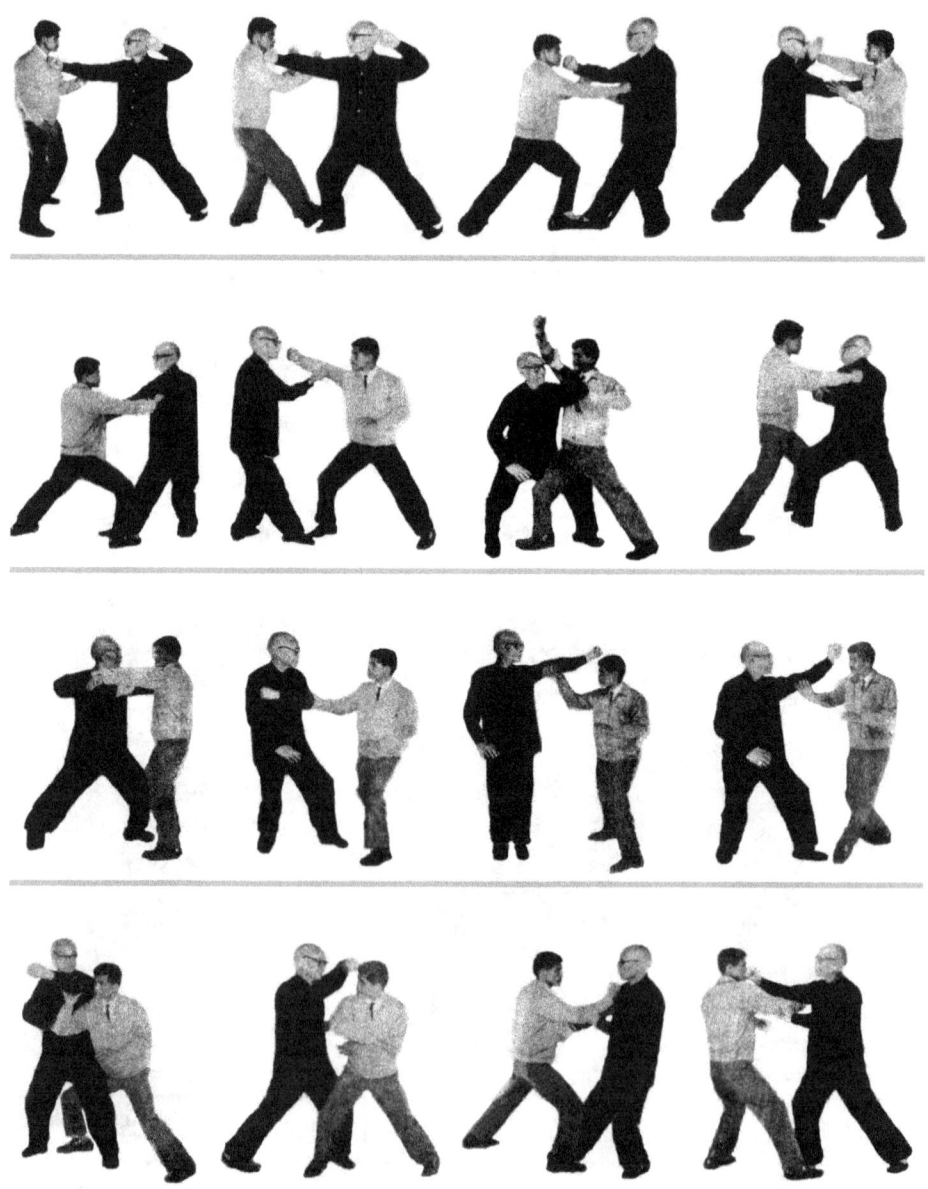

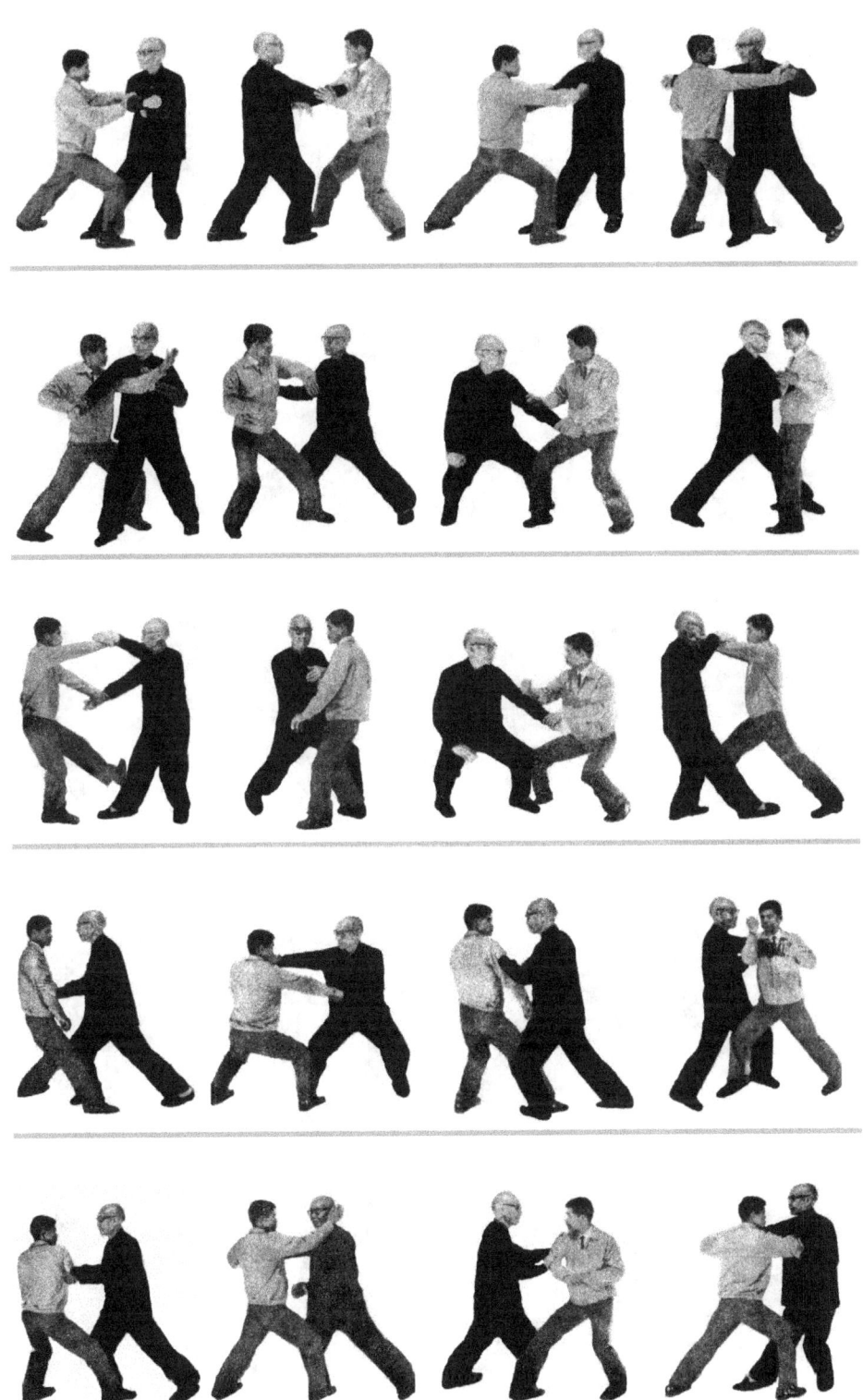

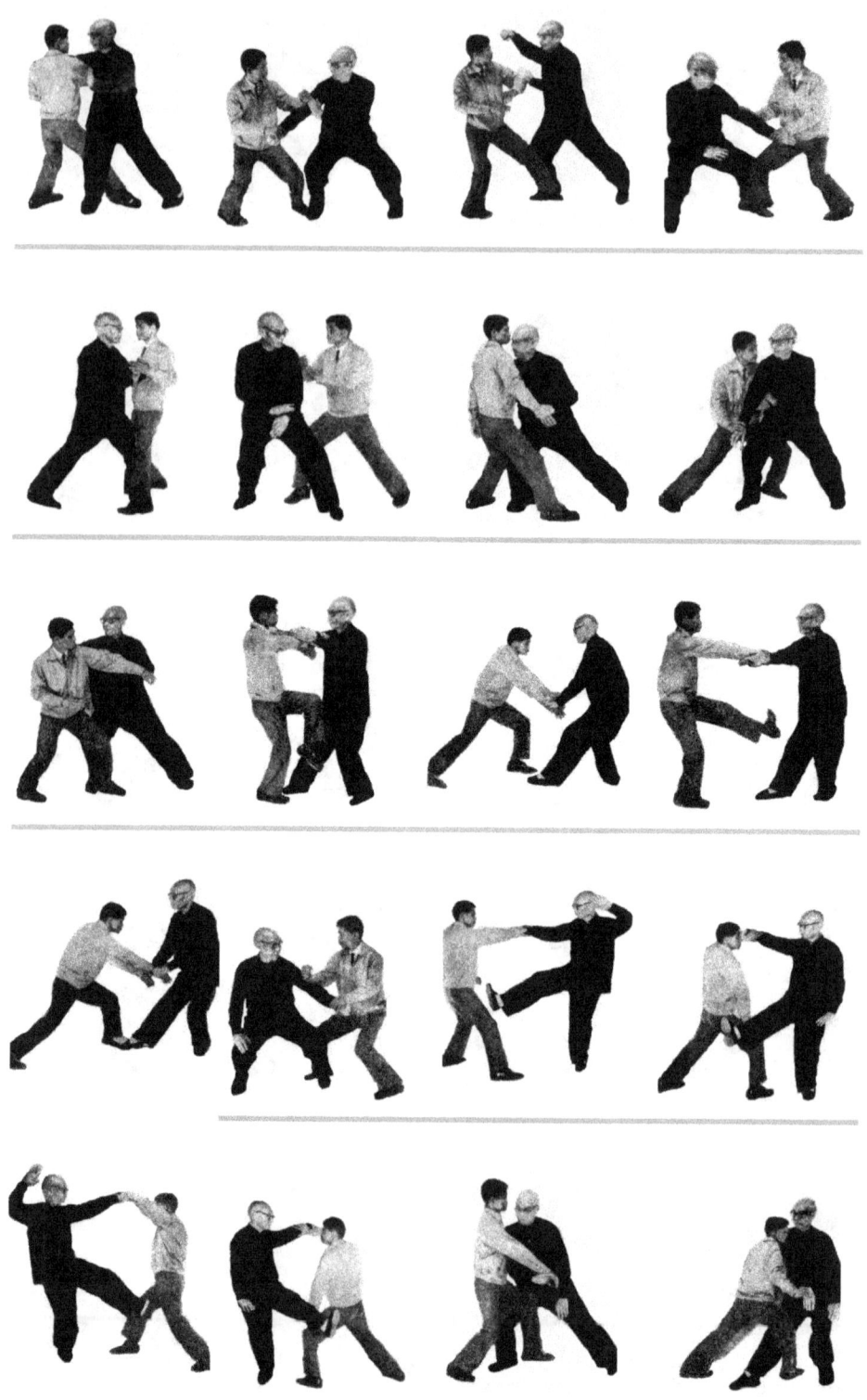

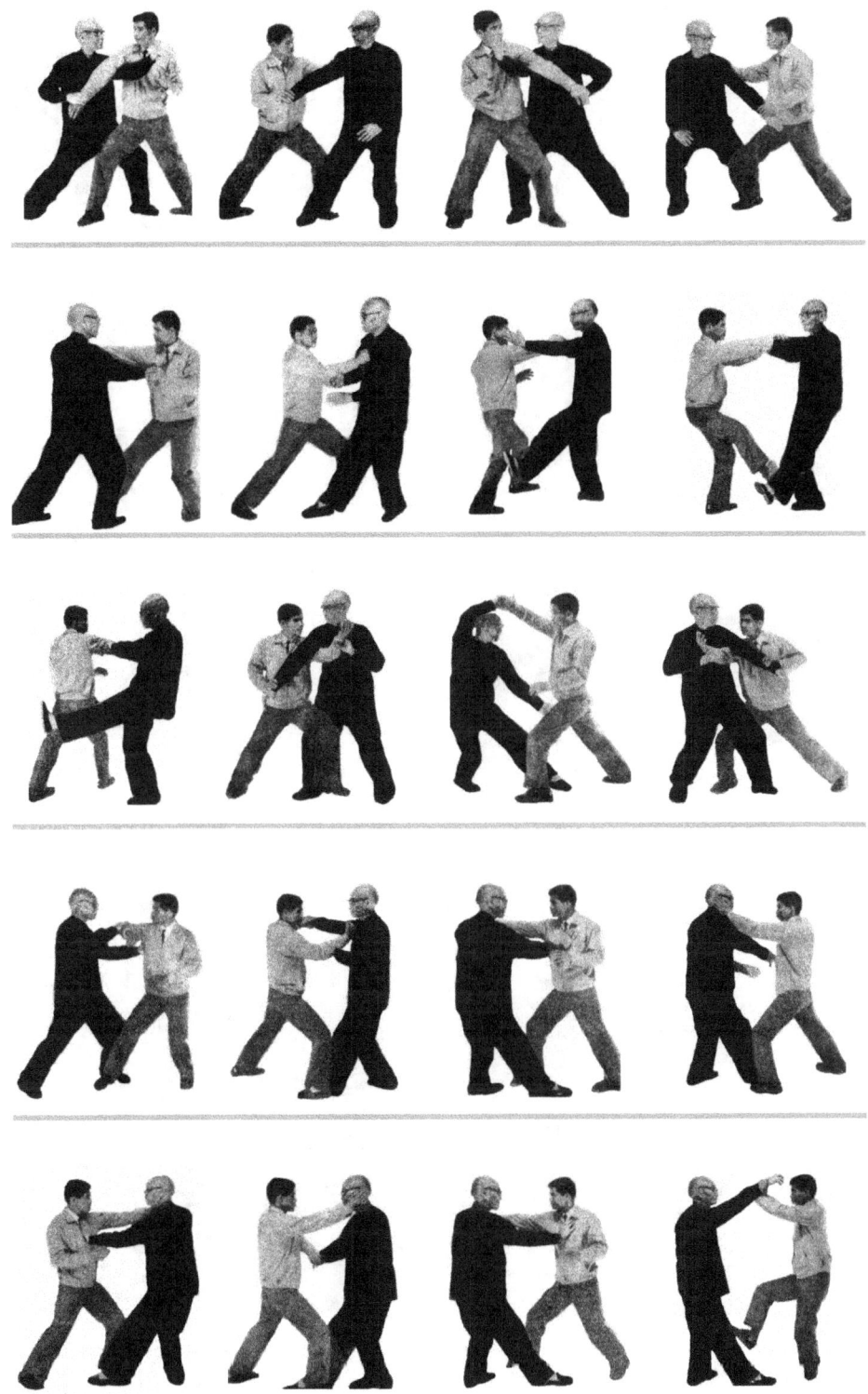

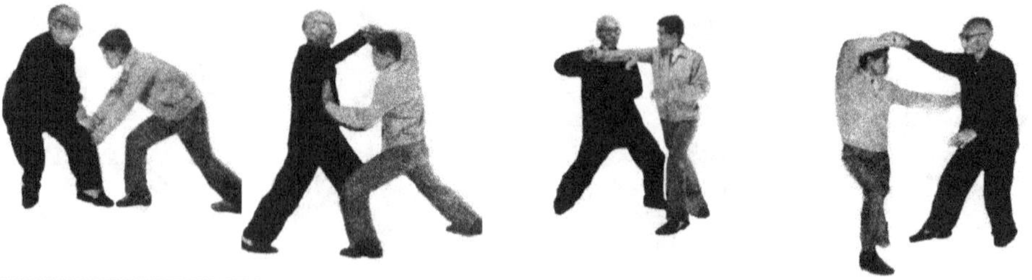

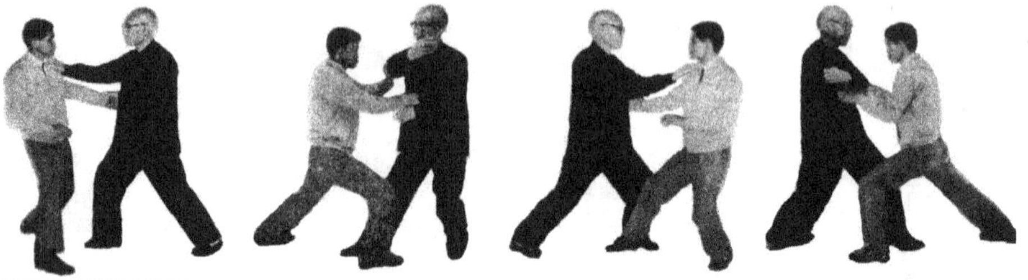

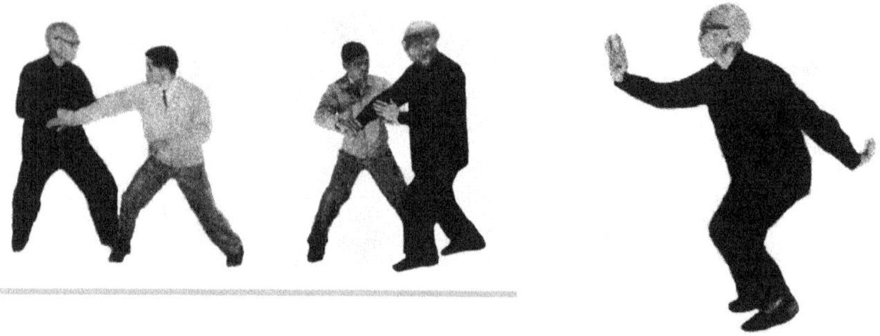

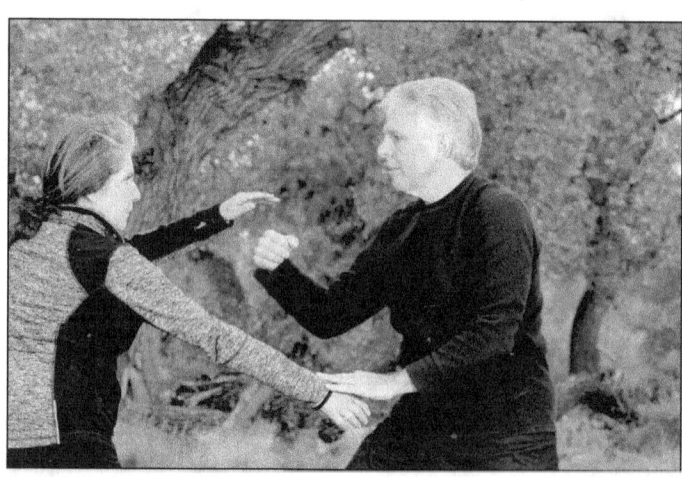

The author and top student Debra Rivera practicing paired sanshou practice, emphasizing the embodyment of taiji principles into practical applications, blending defense with attack.

6

Taiji Straight Sword Routines (solo/paired)

Master Xiong wrote a book titled *Illustrated Guide to Tai Chi Sword Techniques*. In it he details each fifty-eight techniques and their applications. It is easy to see that the form is Yang Style and follows the fundamental forms and principles embodied in the taiji solo routine.

From numerous photographs and videos of Yang Style sword forms, there is a continuity of style and function. The heritage is also based on Xiong's autobiography, information from the Zhirou Quan Society ("soft boxing society") founded by Chen Weiming, and the preface written by Hu Pu'an in Chen's *Taiji Sword* (1927) book. Xiong's single sword routine is clearly inherited through a lineage of instruction. The lineage is as follows:

Yang Luchan (1799-1872)	*This chart*
▼	*is mainly*
Yang Jianhou (1839-1917)	*that of*
▼	*Hu Pu'an.*
Yang Chengfu (1883-1936)	*To clarify,*
▼	*Xiong studied*
Chen Weiming (1881-1958)	*directly under*
▼	*a number of*
Hu Pu'an (1878-1947)	*teachers,*
▼	*particularly*
Xiong Yanghe (1888-1981)	*Yang Jianhou.*

There are some quality books and videos available on the taiji straight sword discussing its history, form and functions. The following pages present Xiong performing the routine. Although Xiong is elderly in these photographs and in his other books, he exhibits fine form that after his decades of practice carried him into his 90s in good health.

1) beginning   起勢
2) advance, unite with sword   上步合劍
3) immortal points the way   仙人指路
4) three rings around the moon   三環套月
5) big dipper   大魁星
6) swallow skims the water   燕子抄水
7) right, block, clear the way   右攔掃
8) left, block, clear the way   左攔掃
9) small dipper   小魁星
10) wasp enters cave   黃蜂入洞
11) nimble cat catches the mouse   靈貓捕鼠
12) dragonfly touches the water   蜻蜓點水
13) swallow returns to the nest   燕子入巢
14) phoenix spreads its wings   鳳凰雙展翅
15) dragonfly touches the water   蜻蜓點水
16) whirlwind (R)   右旋風
17) small dipper   小魁星
18) embrace the moon   懷中抱月
19) whirlwind (L)   左旋風
20) waiting like a fish   等魚式
21) poke the grass in search of a snake   撥草尋蛇
22) embrace the moon   懷中抱月
23) send the bird to the forest   送鳥上林
24) dark dragon waves its tail   烏龍擺尾
25) rolling wind sweeps lotus leaves   風捲荷葉
26) lion shakes its head   獅子搖頭
27) tiger carries its head   虎抱頭
28) wild horse jumps the ravine   野馬跳澗
29) turnover, rein in the horse   翻身勒馬
30) compass needle points south   指南針
31) meeting wind and dust   迎風撣塵
32) push the boat with the current   順水推舟
33) meteor chases the moon   流星趕月
34) heavenly bird descends like a waterfall   天鳥飛瀑
35) lift the curtain   挑簾式
36) wheel the sword left and right   左右車輪劍

37) swallow holds the mud 燕子啣泥
38) mythic bird; spreads its wings 大鵬展翅
39) scoop up the moon from the sea bottom 海底撈月
40) embrace the moon 懷中抱月
41) the nature spirit (Yaksha) explores the sea 夜叉探海
42) rhinoceros gazes at the moon 犀牛望月
43) shoot the wild goose 射雁式
44) green dragon extends its talons 青龍探爪
45) phoenix spreads its wings 鳳凰雙展翅
46) cross over the hurdle (L) 左跨欄
47) cross over the hurdle (R) 右跨欄
48) shoot the wild goose 射雁式
49) white ape offers fruit 白猿獻果
50) falling flowers 落花式
51) jade lady threads the shuttle 玉女穿梭
52) white tiger stirs its tail 白虎攬尾
53) fish leaps over dragon gate 魚躍龍門
54) dark dragon twists around a post 烏龍絞柱
55) immortal points the way 仙人指路
56) wind sweeps the plum blossoms 風掃梅花
57) hold the ivory ancestral tablet 手捧牙笏
58) embrace the sword, return to original posture 抱劍歸原

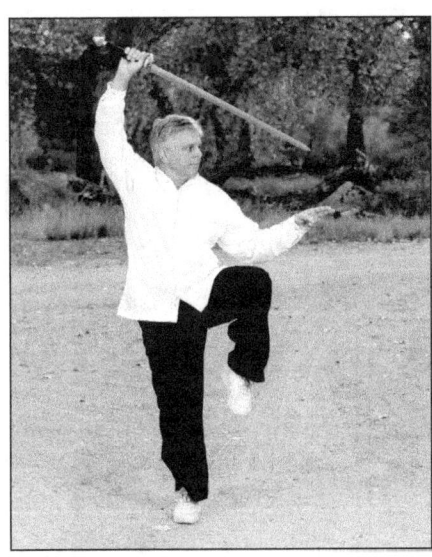
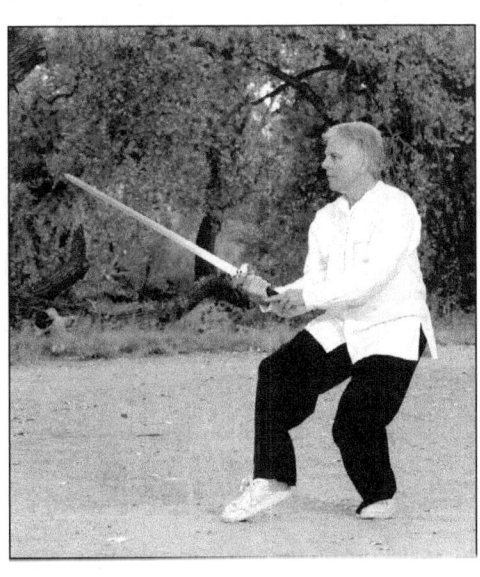

The author trying his best to grasp Xiong's taijji straight sword routine.

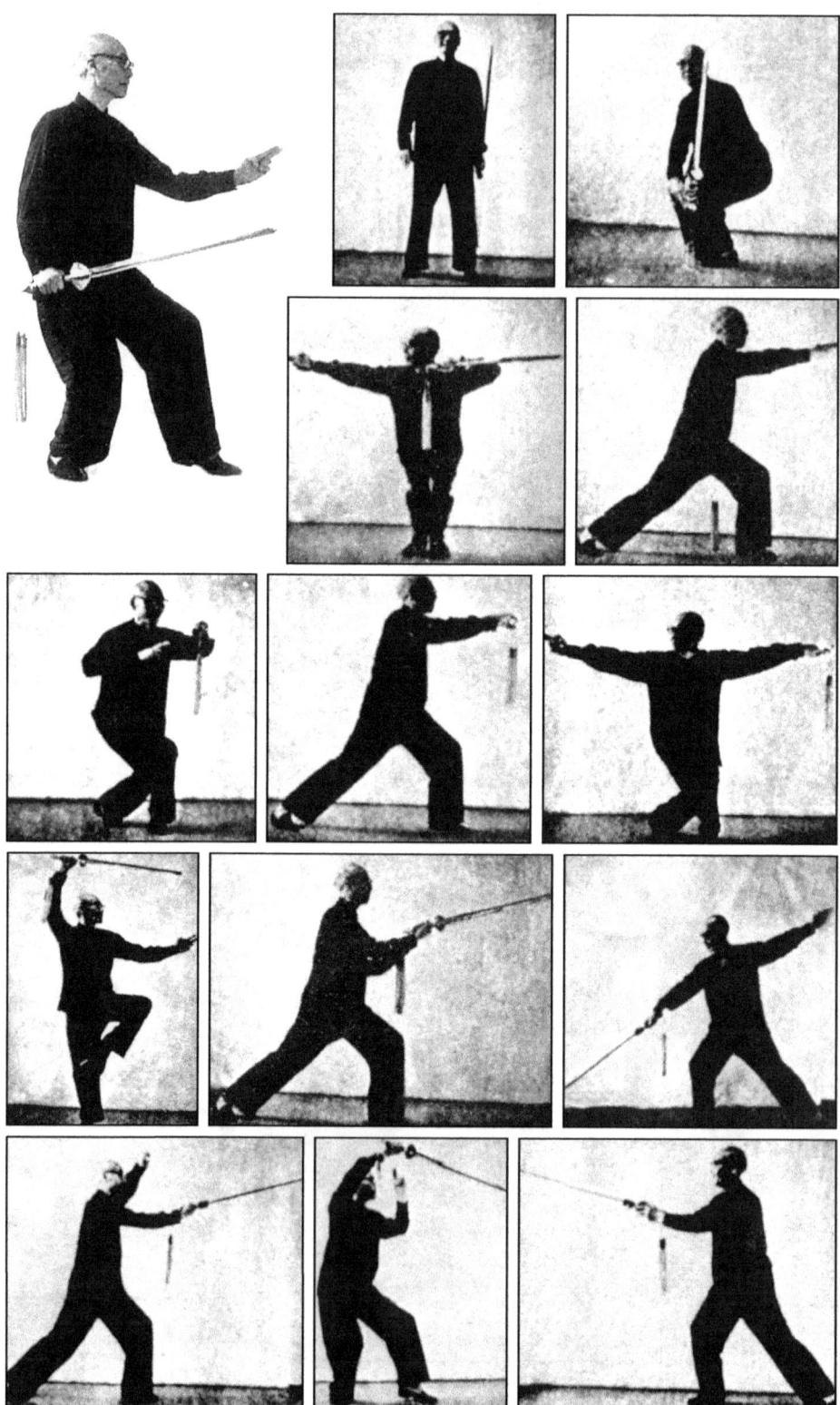

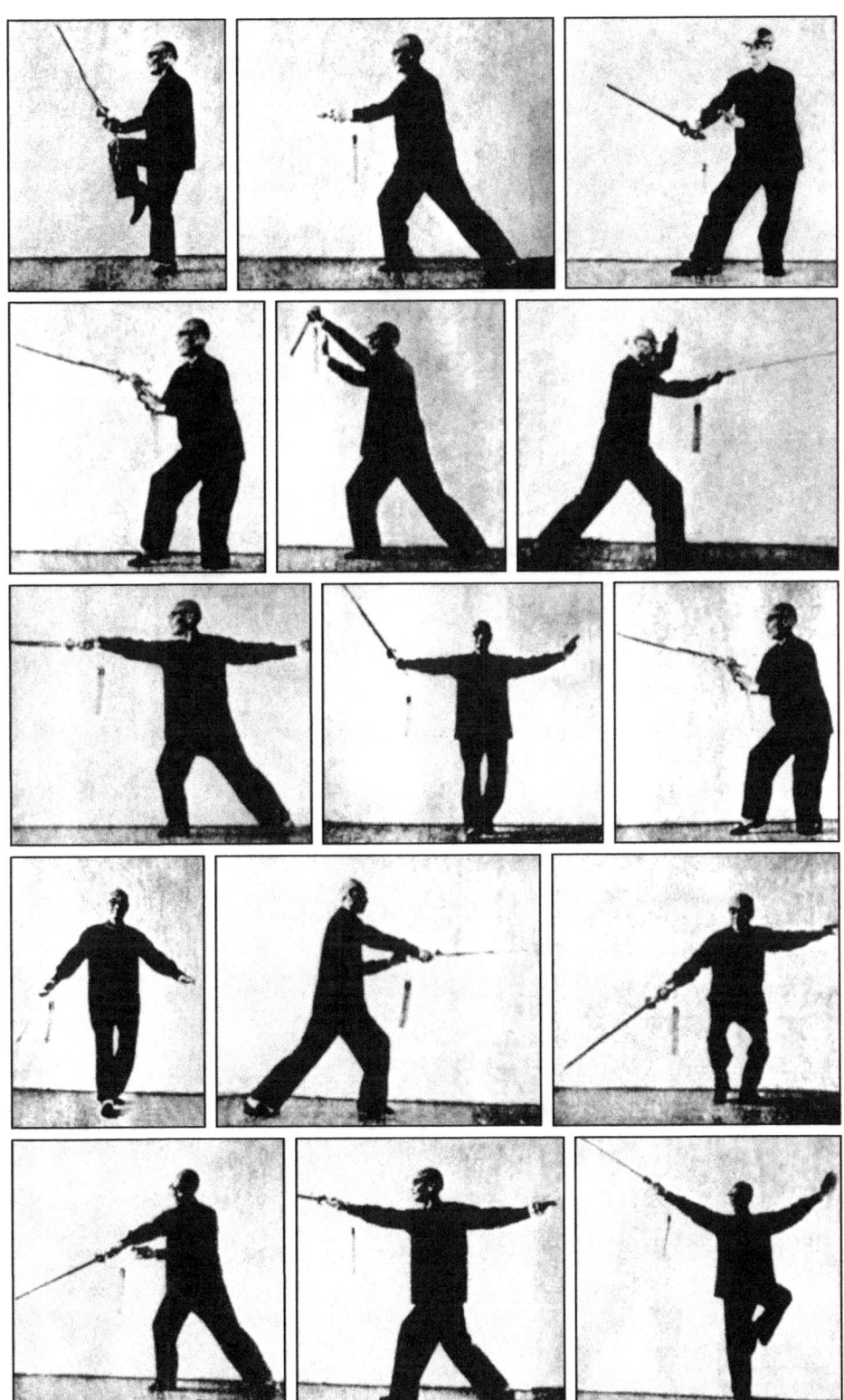

49

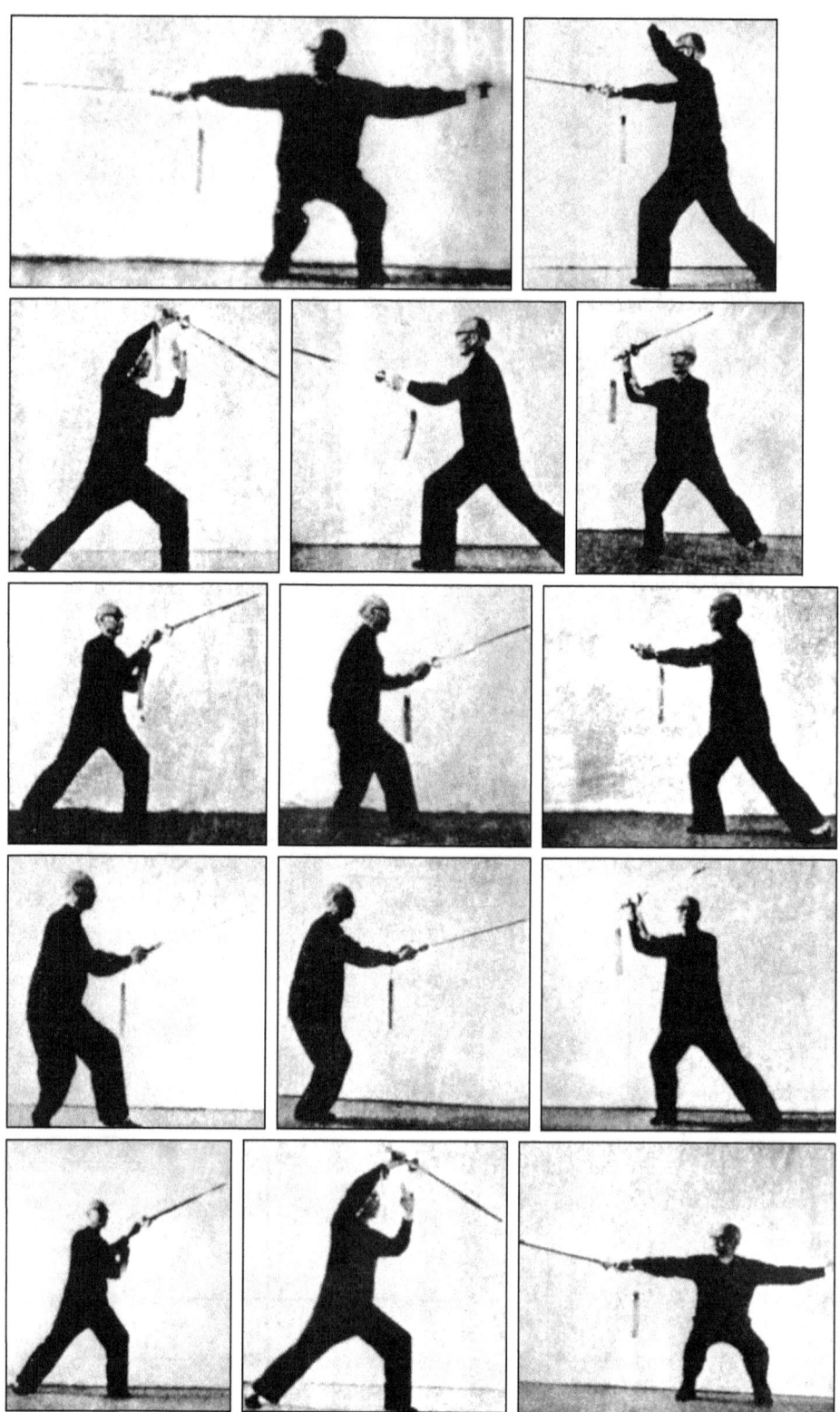

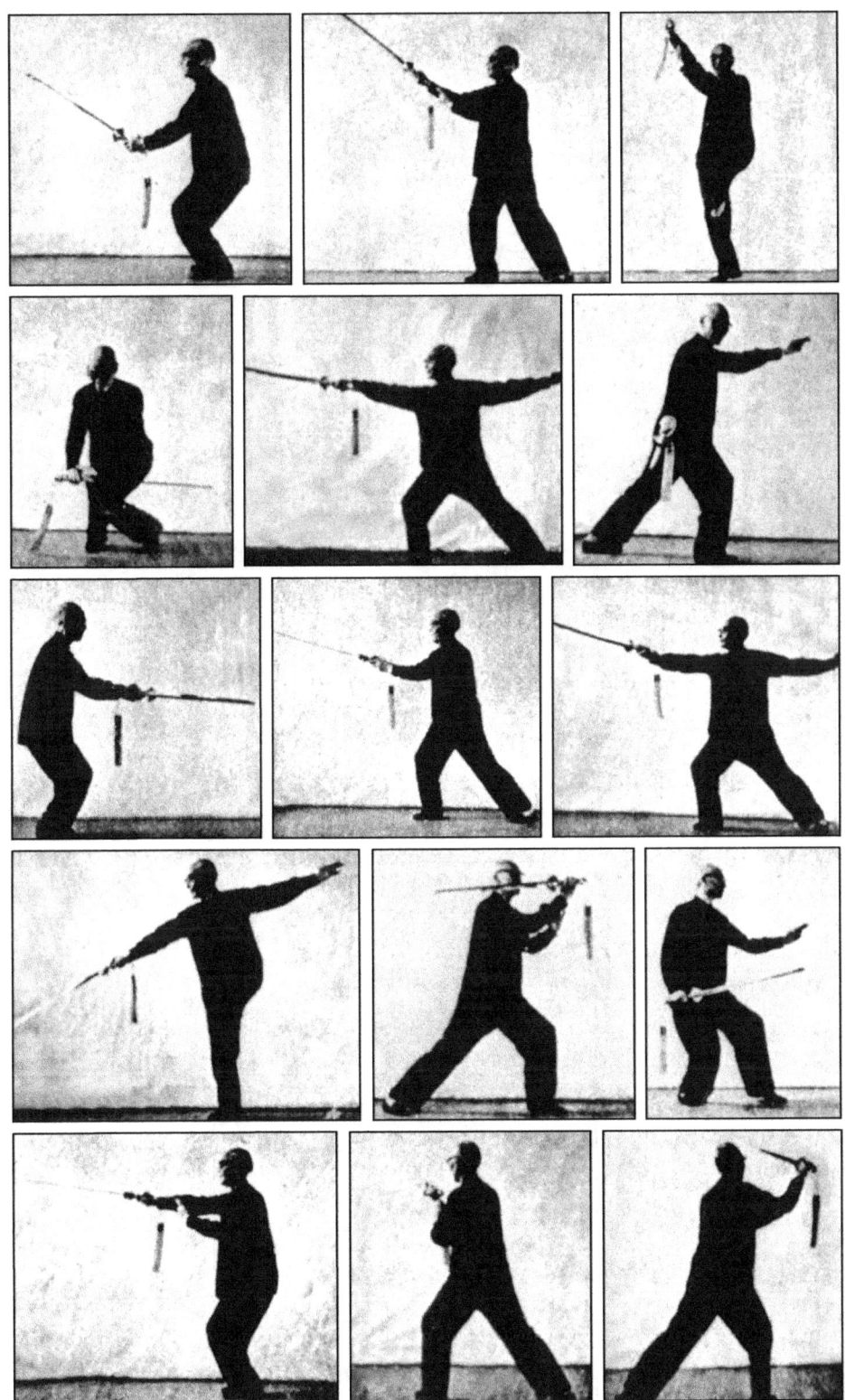

51

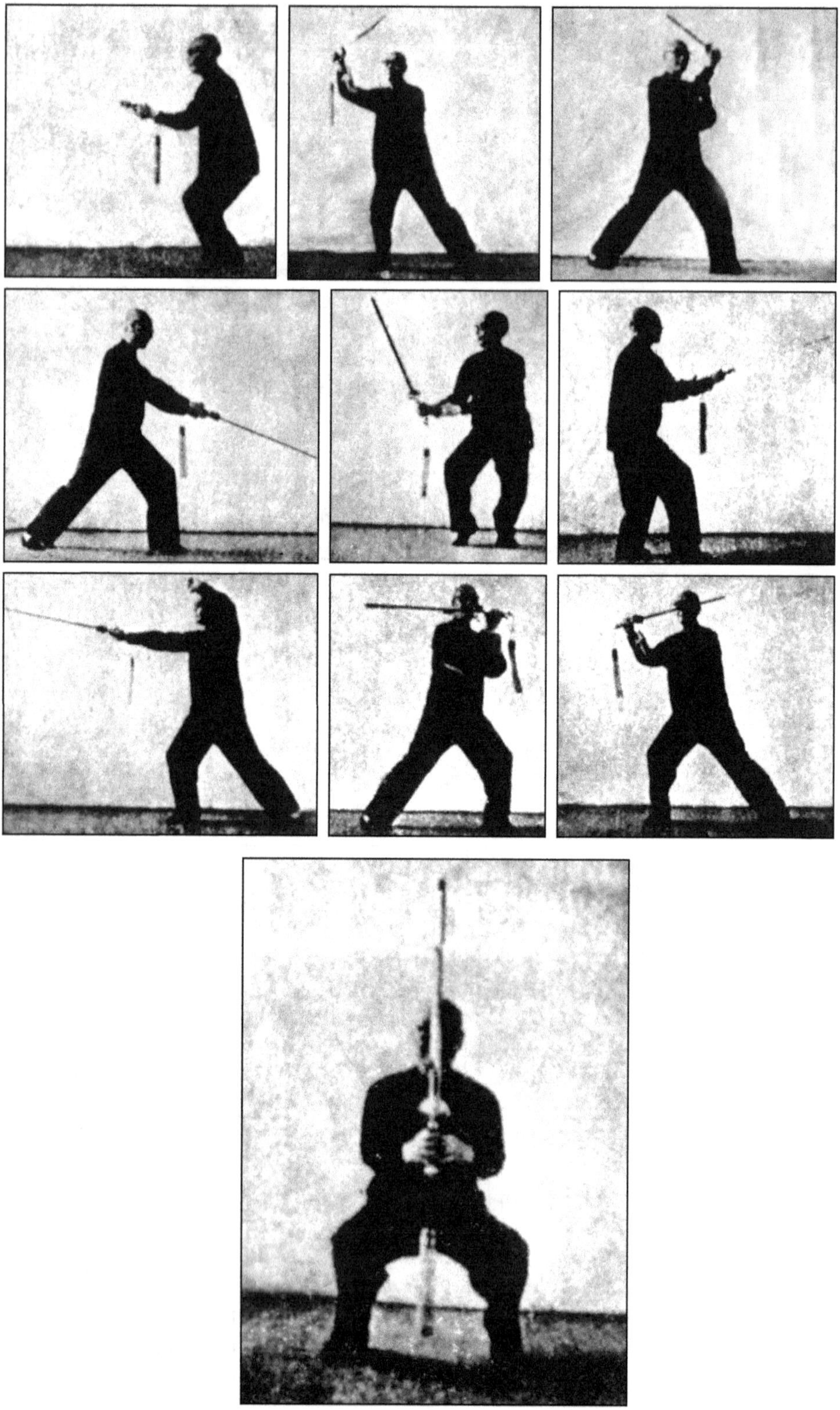

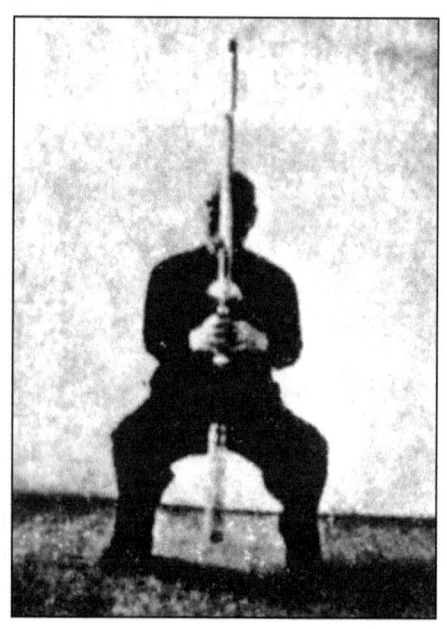

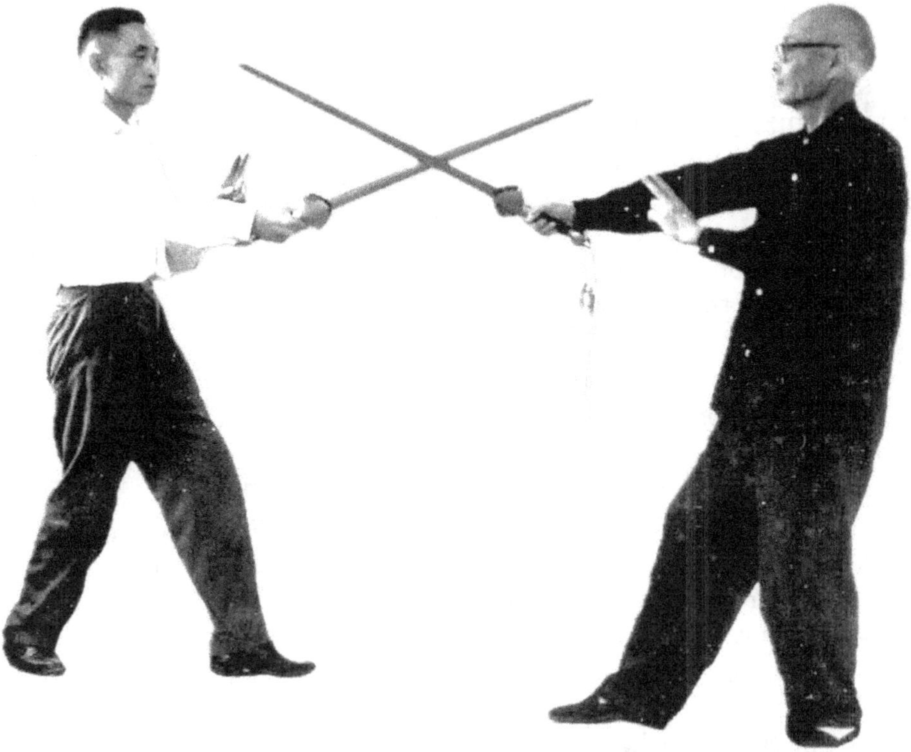

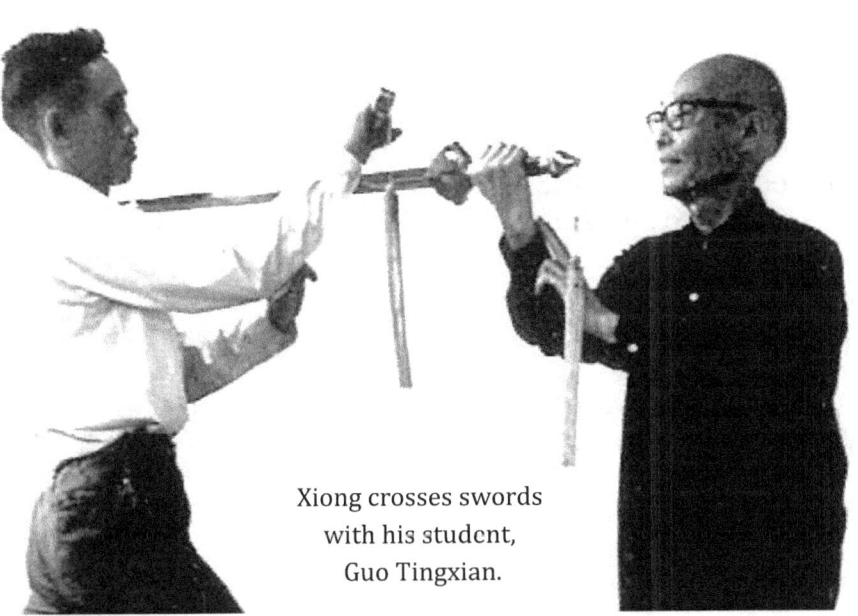

Xiong crosses swords
with his student,
Guo Tingxian.

1) beginning 起勢
2) immortal points the way 仙人指路
3) cross swords 交劍式
4) wasp enters the cave 黃蜂入洞
5) small dipper 小魁星
6) phoenix spreads both wings 鳳凰雙展翅
7) shoot the wild goose 射雁式
8) advance and chop 進步劈
9) paired retreat and advance (twice) 對提先退後進各兩次
10) circle around, change step 繞走換步
11) embrace the moon 懷中抱月
12) left block, sweep 左攔掃
13) right cross block 右跨攔
14) phoenix spreads both wings 鳳凰雙展翅
15) white tiger stirs its tail, advance, retreat 白虎攬尾,先進後退
16) paired chopping 對劈
17) right whirlwind (twice) 右旋風-兩次
18) left whirlwind (twice) 左旋風-兩次
19) right wrap, left turn 右絞左轉
20) dragon returns, right block, sweep 迴龍右攔掃
21) rhinoceros gazes at the moon 犀牛望月
22) right cross block, mythic bird spreads wings 右跨攔大鵬展翅
23) right cross block, right parry 右跨攔, 右撥式
24) shoot the wild goose 射雁式
25) step forward, left block, sweep 進步左攔掃
26) shoot the wild goose 射雁式
27) nature spirit explores the sea 夜叉探海
28) swallow returns to nest 燕子入巢
29) shoot the wild goose 射雁式
30) mythic bird spreads its wings 大鵬展翅
31) black dragon waves its tail 烏龍擺尾
32) wind sweeps lotus leaves 風捲荷葉
33) right cross block 右跨攔
34) left cross block 左跨攔
35) black dragon waves its tail 烏龍擺尾
36) search for snake in grass, retreat, advance 撥草尋蛇, 先退後進
37) wrist circling thrust, retreat, advance 運腕撥刺,先退後進
38) send the bird to the forest 送鳥上林
39) shoot the wild goose 射雁式
40) cross swords, return to original posture 交劍歸原

1) beginning　　　　　　　　　　　　　　　　起勢
2) immortal points the way　　　　　　　　　仙人指路
3) cross swords　　　　　　　　　　　　　　交劍式
4) wasps enter the cave　　　　　　　　　　黃蜂入洞
5) small dipper　　　　　　　　　　　　　　小魁星
6) right sweep block (brush dust in the wind) 右跨攔 （迎風撢塵）
7) shooting the wild goose　　　　　　　　　射雁式
8) step back, raise sword (linking transition) 退步提,連接下式
9) paired advance and retreat (twice)　　　對提,先進後退各兩次
10) circle around and change step　　　　　繞走換步
11) left sweep block　　　　　　　　　　　　左跨攔
12) embrace the moon　　　　　　　　　　　懷中抱月
13) black dragon wags its tail　　　　　　　烏龍 擺尾
14) wind scatters lotus leaves, bird flies to forest 風捲荷葉送鳥上林
15) white tiger flicks its tail; retreat, advance 白虎攪尾,先退後進
16) paired chop　　　　　　　　　　　　　　對劈
17) left whirlwind (twice)　　　　　　　　　左 旋風,兩次
18) right whirlwind (twice)　　　　　　　　右 旋風,兩次
19) left twist, follow, turning sweep block　左絞隨轉左攔掃
20) right wheel sword　　　　　　　　　　　右車輪劍
21) right sweep block (brush dust in the wind) 右跨攔 （迎風撢塵）
22) relax left, advance and right chop　　　左鬆右進劈
23) little immortal star, step back　　　　　小魁星,退步
24) shoot the wild goose　　　　　　　　　射雁式
25) neutralize right, advance with left chop　右化左進劈
26) shoot the wild goose　　　　　　　　　射雁式
27) nature spirit explores the sea　　　　　夜叉探海
28) swallows returns to nest　　　　　　　燕子入巢
29) shoot the wild goose　　　　　　　　　射雁式
30) relax left, chop right　　　　　　　　　左鬆右劈
31) right wheel sword　　　　　　　　　　　右車輪劍
32) right sweep block, step forward with left 右跨攔-跟進左步
33) left sweep block　　　　　　　　　　　　左跨攔
34) right sweep block　　　　　　　　　　　右跨攔
35) part grass search for snake, advance, retreat 撥草尋蛇,先進後退
36) wrist circling thrust, advance, retreat　運腕撥刺,先進後退
37) lift the curtain　　　　　　　　　　　　挑簾式
38) deflect right　　　　　　　　　　　　　右撥式
39) shoot the wild goose　　　　　　　　　射雁式
40) return to original posture　　　　　　　交劍歸原

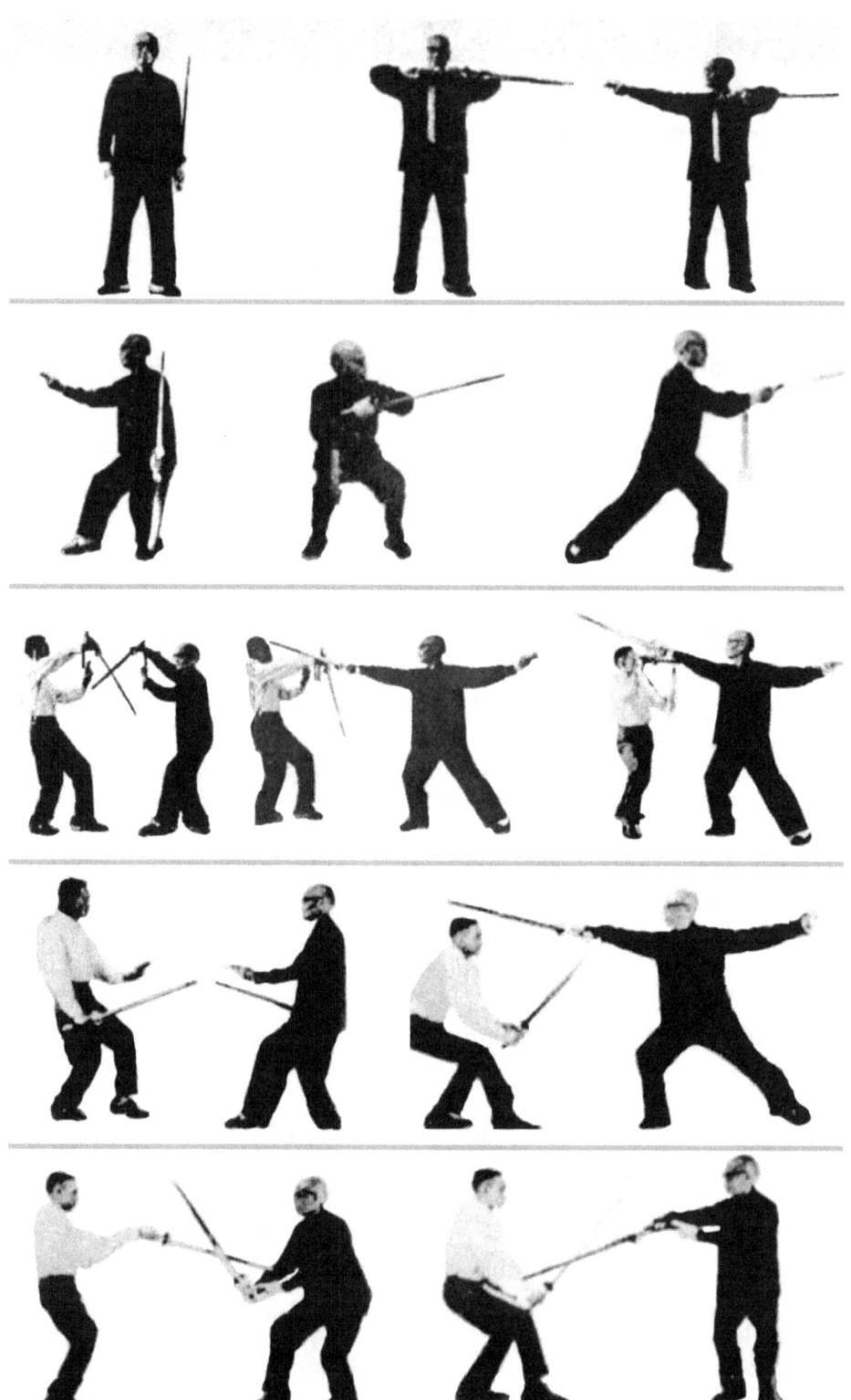

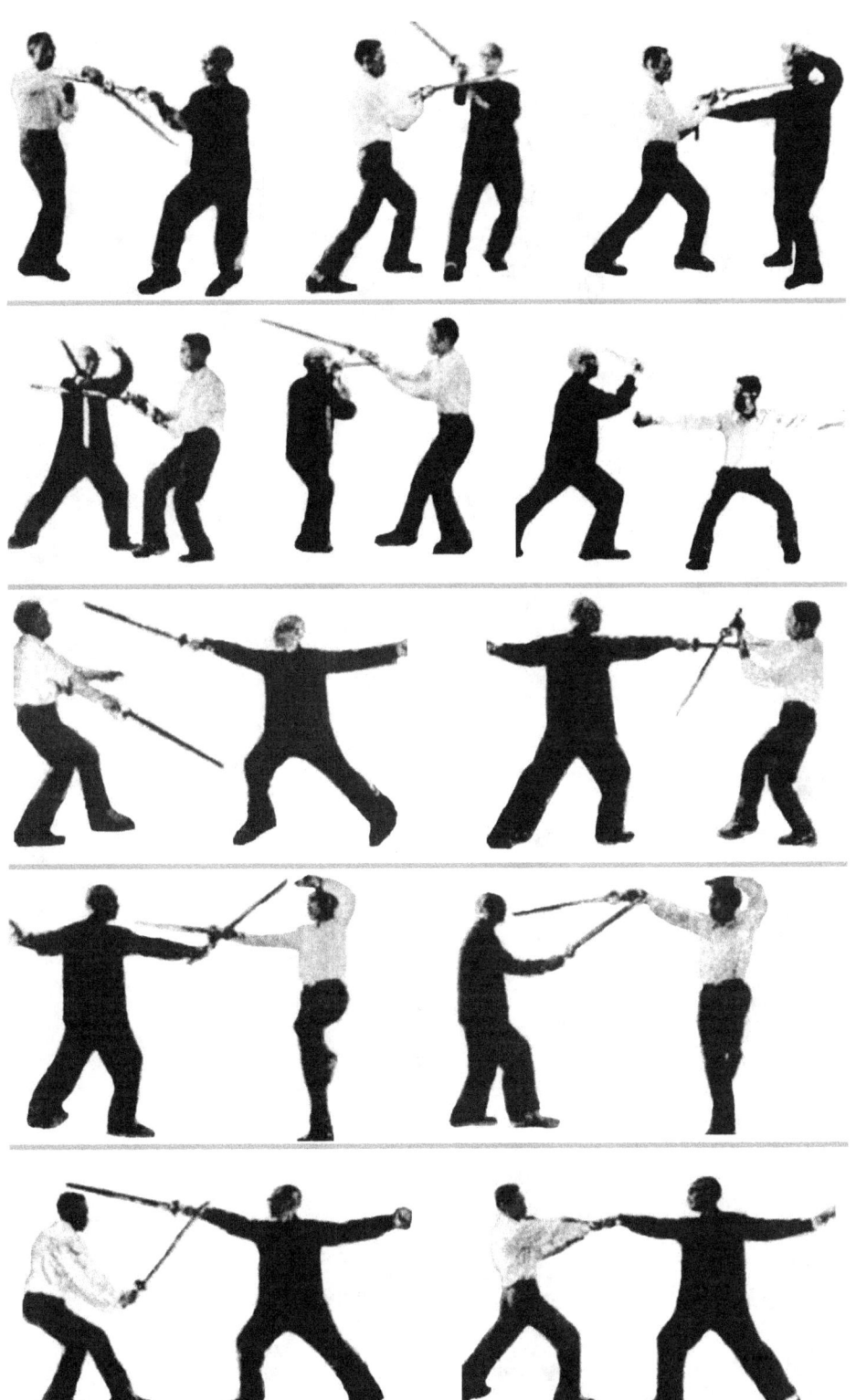

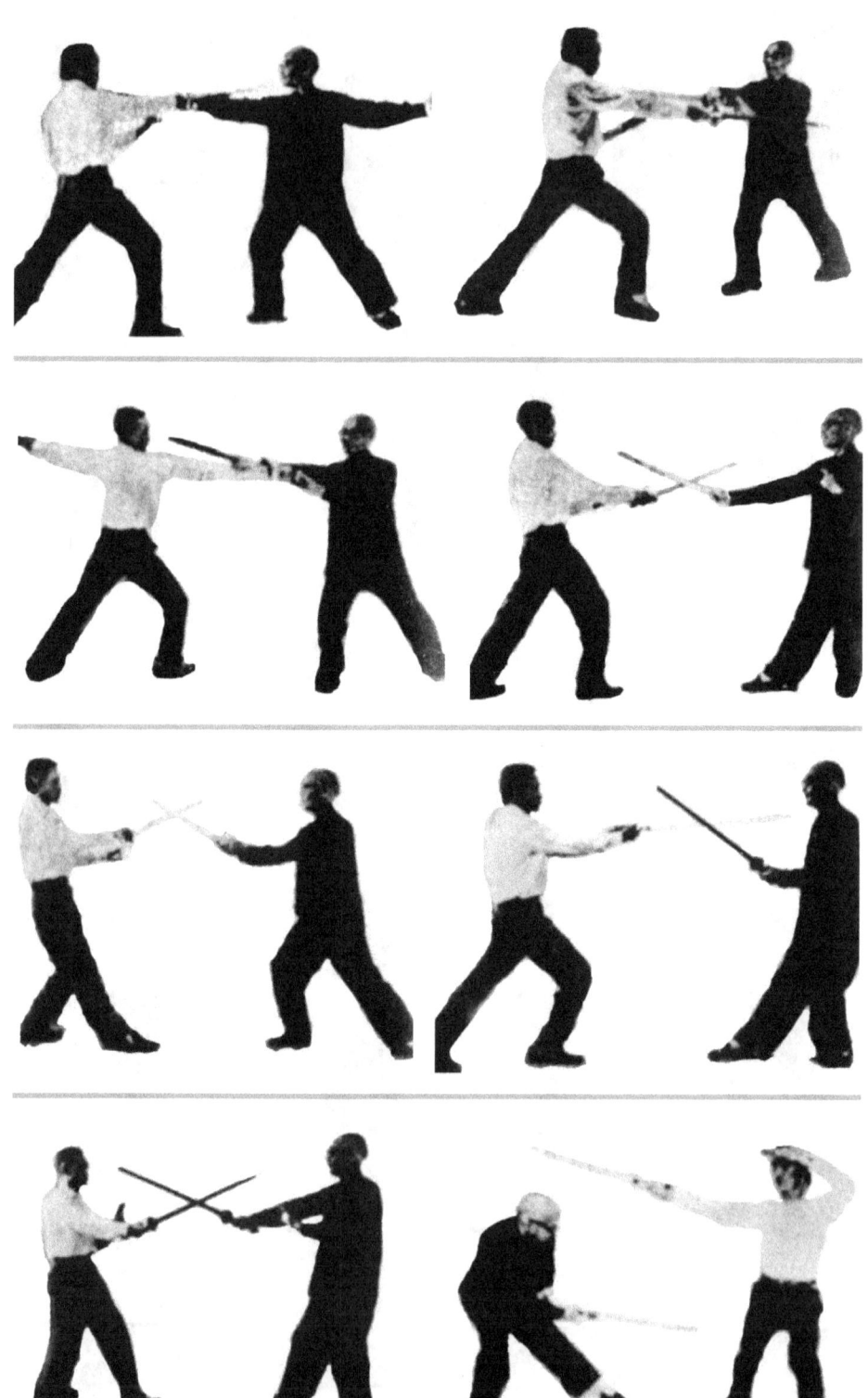

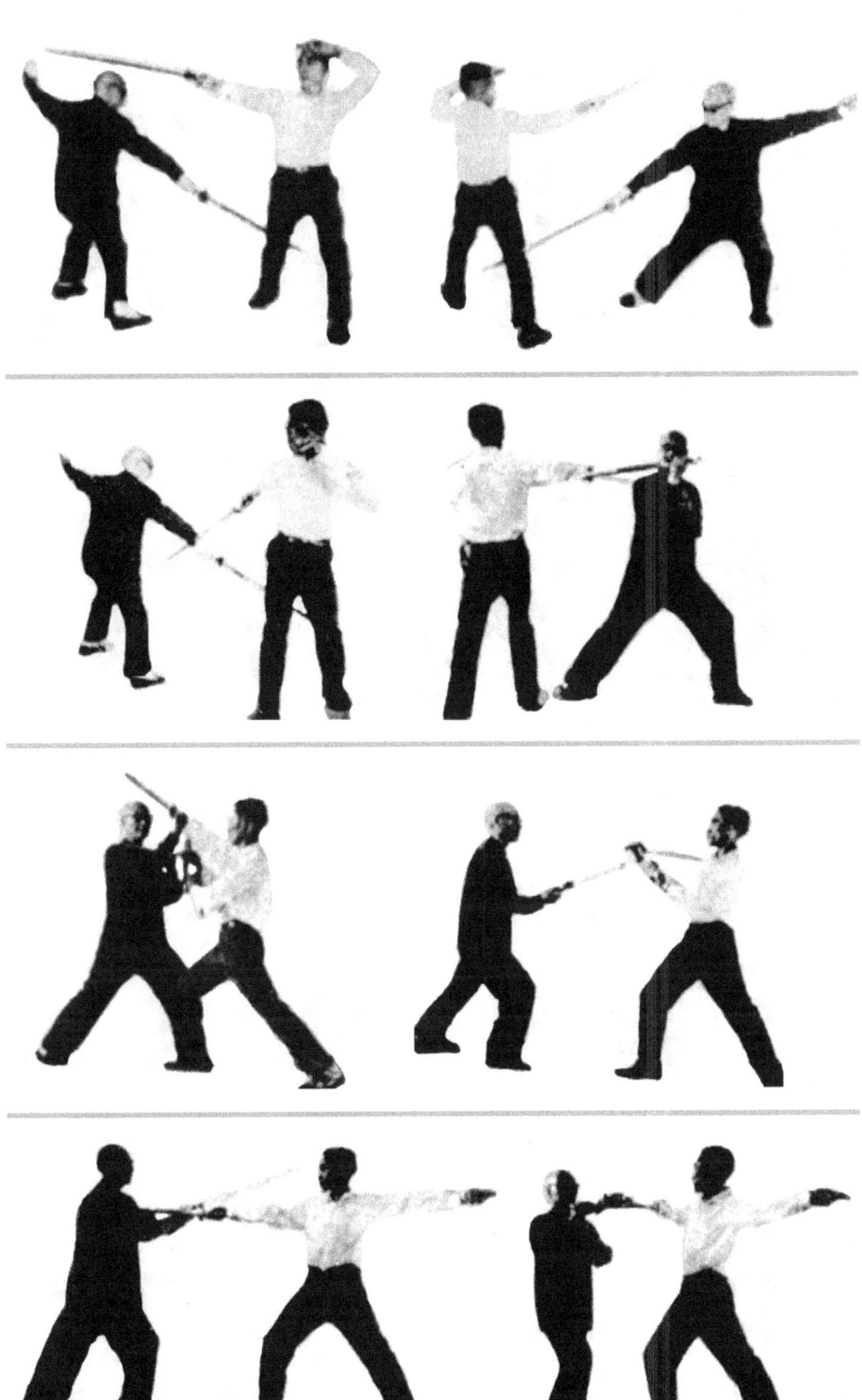

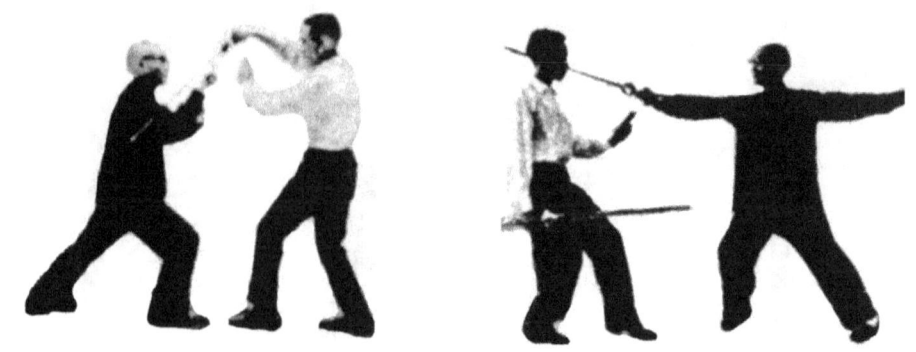

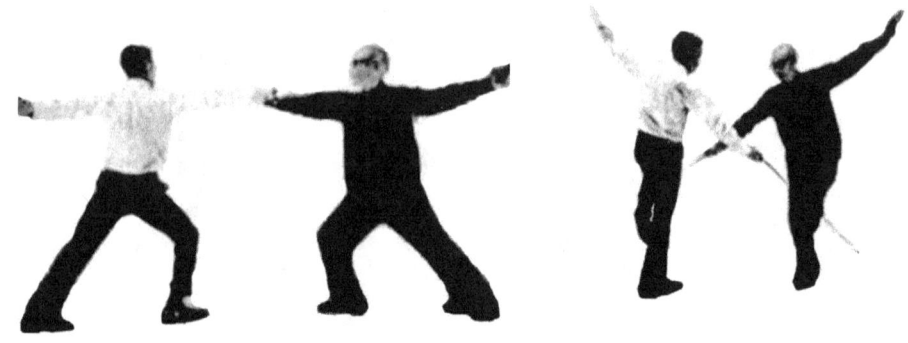

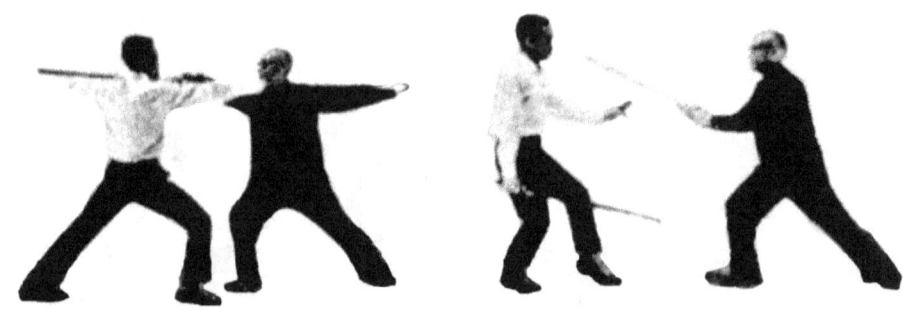

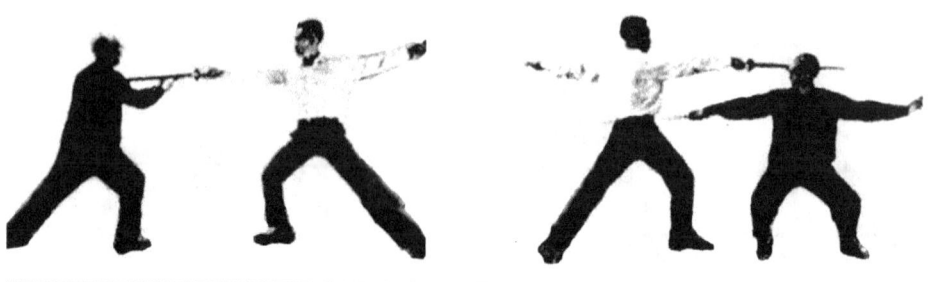

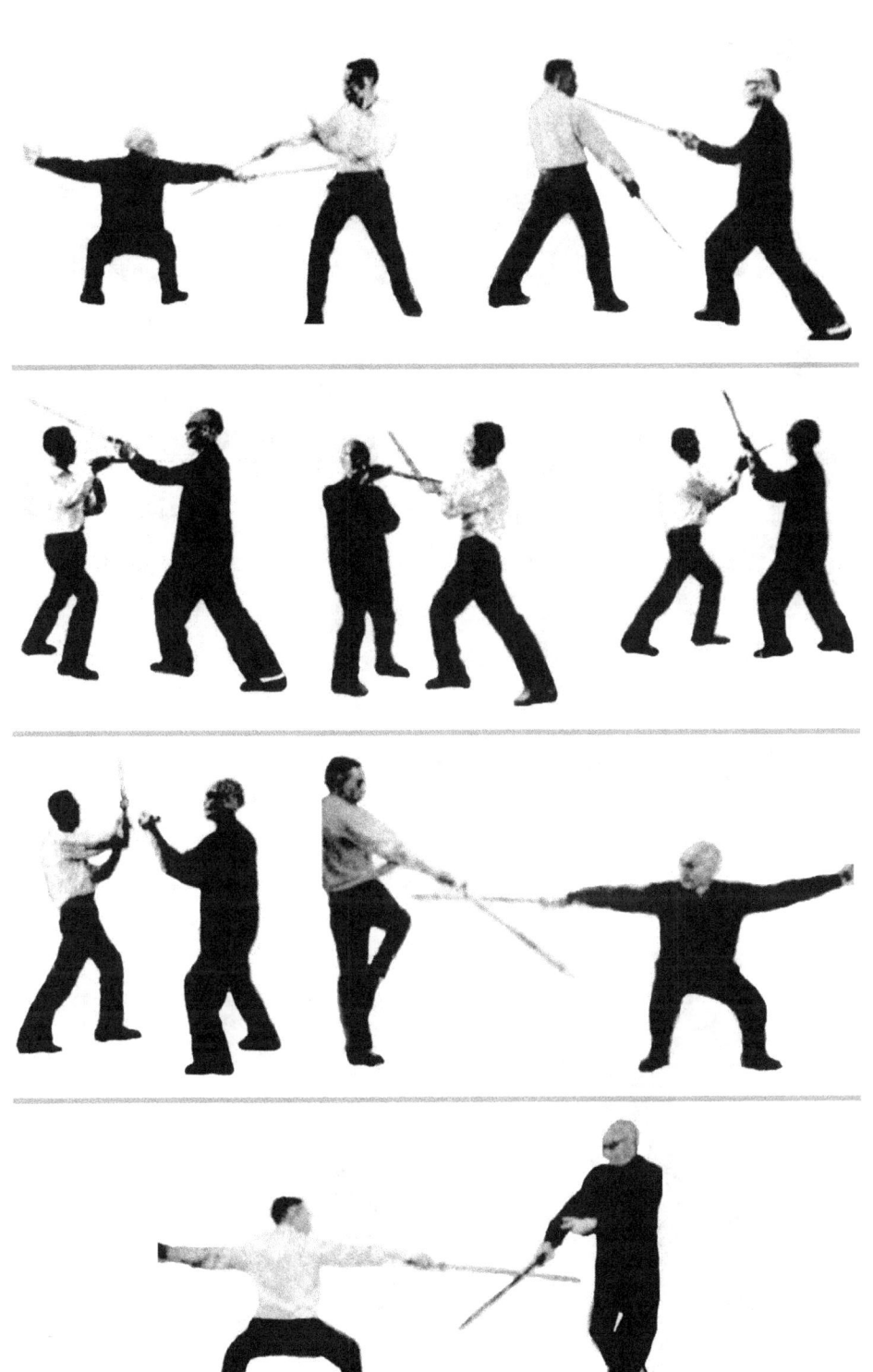

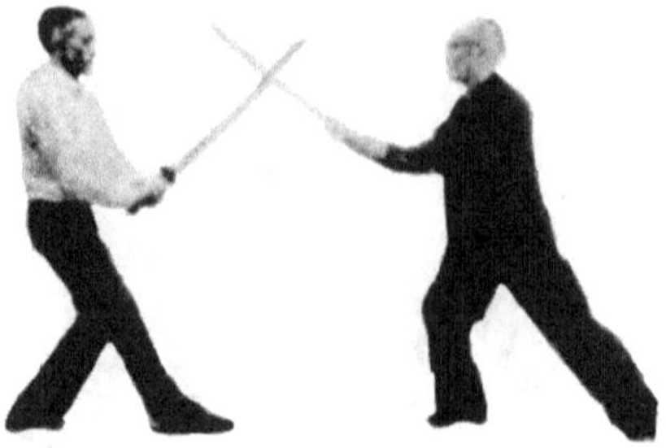

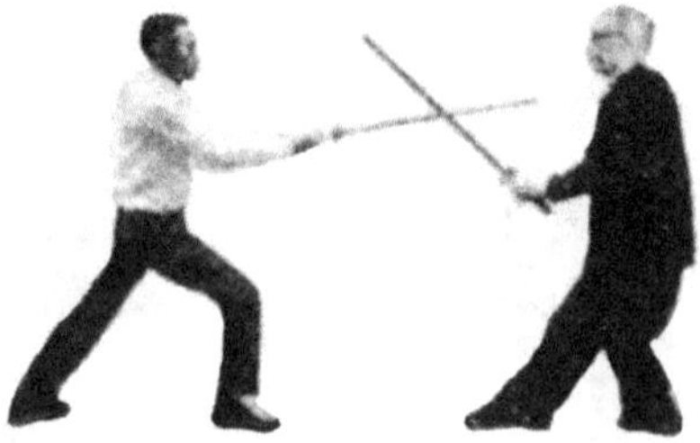

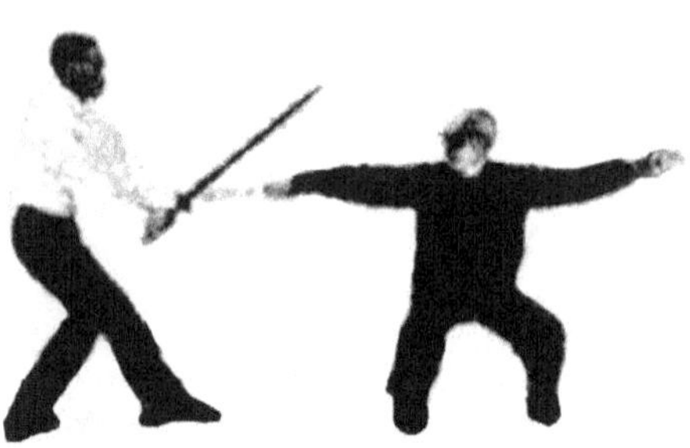

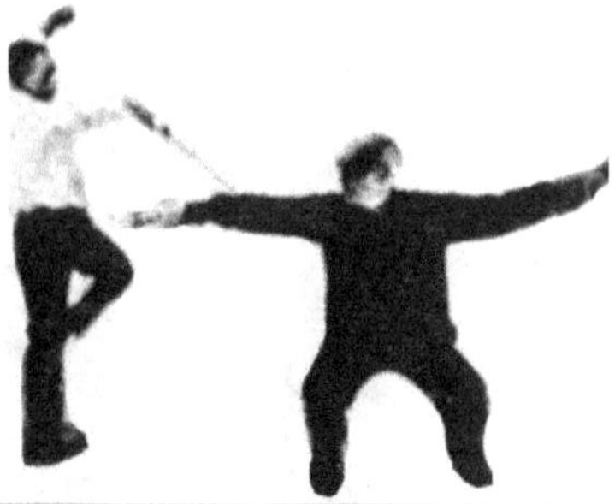

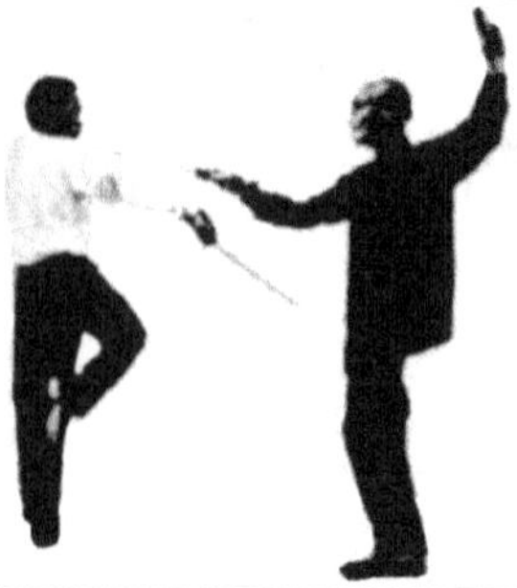

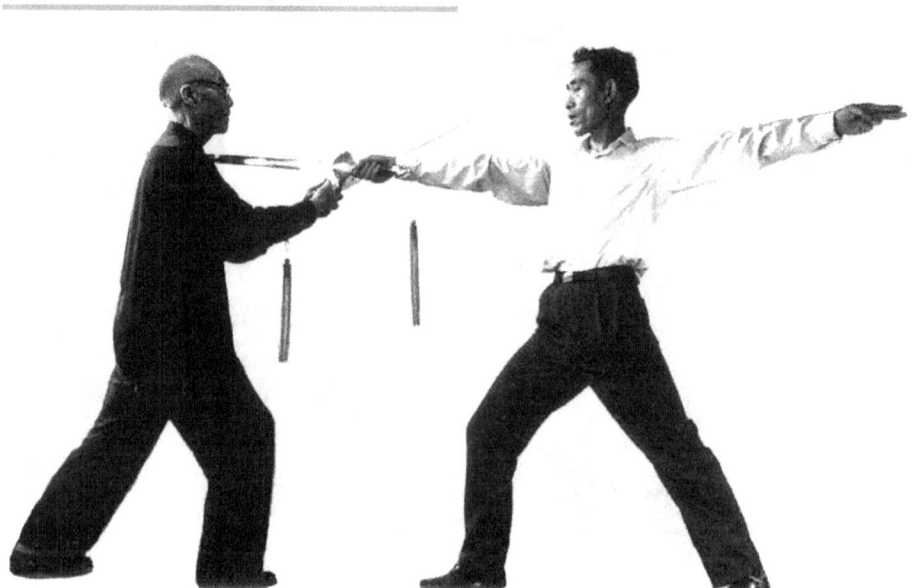

7

Taiji Broadsword Routines (solo/paired)

The solo broadsword routine consists of thirty-three movements. Unlike the straight sword with two sharp sides, the curved broadsword is only sharp on one side. The shape of the weapon affects how techniques are applied, and the practitioner can feel a difference in the body movement when practicing with each sword type. Weapons are manipulated according to their characteristics, being long or short, curved or straight. Straight weapons focus on thrusting while curved weapons are feature cutting techniques.

The solo broadsword form is basic, but it prepares one for the paired routine practice. Movements for the paired sides are numbered forty-one and forty. It's notable that Xiong taught paired routines for various weapons, including the straight sword, broadsword, short staff, and long staff. Many teachers do not know or teach paired routines, so students miss aspects important for self-defense, such as proper distancing and other skills that improve how applications are executed defensively and offensively. Of course, the two-person practices of push hands and dispersing hands were developed for the same purpose.

It has been stated that China has four major weapons: the straight sword (*jian*), long staff (*gun*), spear (*qiang*), and the broadsword (*dao*). The broadsword was very common among soldiers and its simplicity and versality proved effective on the battlefield earning it the nickname of "General of all weapons." The straight sword is often called the "the gentleman of weapons," no doubt because it was favored by scholars. The spear is called the "king of weapons." The long staff is called the "grandfather of all weapons," a fitting description since the long staff/spear is the oldest of weapons.

General Qi Jiguang (1528-1588) taught in Chen Village where taijiquan originated. He would have stressed the four major weapons as Master Xiong had done over his decades teaching.

1) beginning posture 起勢

2) step forward to seven stars 上步七星

3) step back, turn left to seven stars 退步左轉七星

4) white crane spreads wings 白鶴掠翅

5) turn around, conceal the sword 轉身藏刀

6) diagonal push with the sword 斜推刀

7) left upward sword cut 左撩刀

8) right upward sword cut 右撩刀

9) straight push with sword 正推刀

10) jade lady threads the shuttle 玉女穿梭

11) level draw 平拉

12) diagonal push with sword 斜推刀

13) turn around, circle head, conceal sword 轉身盤頭藏刀

14) left sweeping cut 左刮

15) right fanning cut 右搧

16) straight push with sword 正推刀

17) turn around, conceal sword 轉身藏刀

18) upward sword cut 撩刀

19) traveling sword 旅刀

20) upward sword cut 撩刀

21) double rising kicks 二起腿

22) retreat, strike the tiger 撤步打虎勢

23) mandarin duck kicks 鴛鴦腿

24) turn around, circle head, conceal sword 轉身盤頭藏刀

25) push boat with the current 順水推舟

26) turn around, conceal sword 轉身藏刀

27) advance step, upward sword cut 上步撩刀

28) jump and chop downward 跳步剁刀

29) split Mount Hua 力劈華山

30) embrace the sword, draw back 抱刀拉帶

31) chop and stab 劈刺刀

32) turn, change step, chop and slice 轉身換步砍剁

33) closing posture 收刀勢

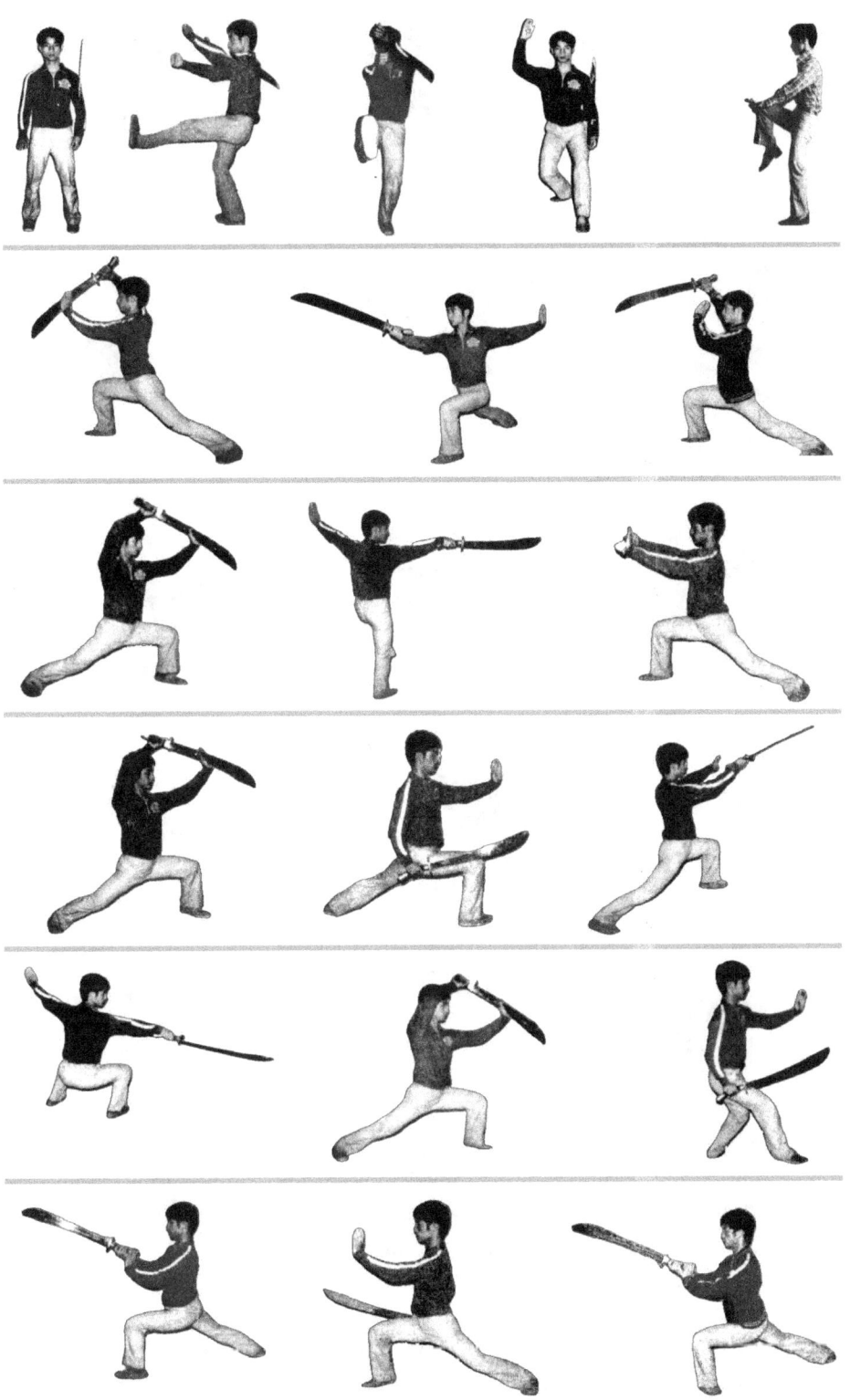

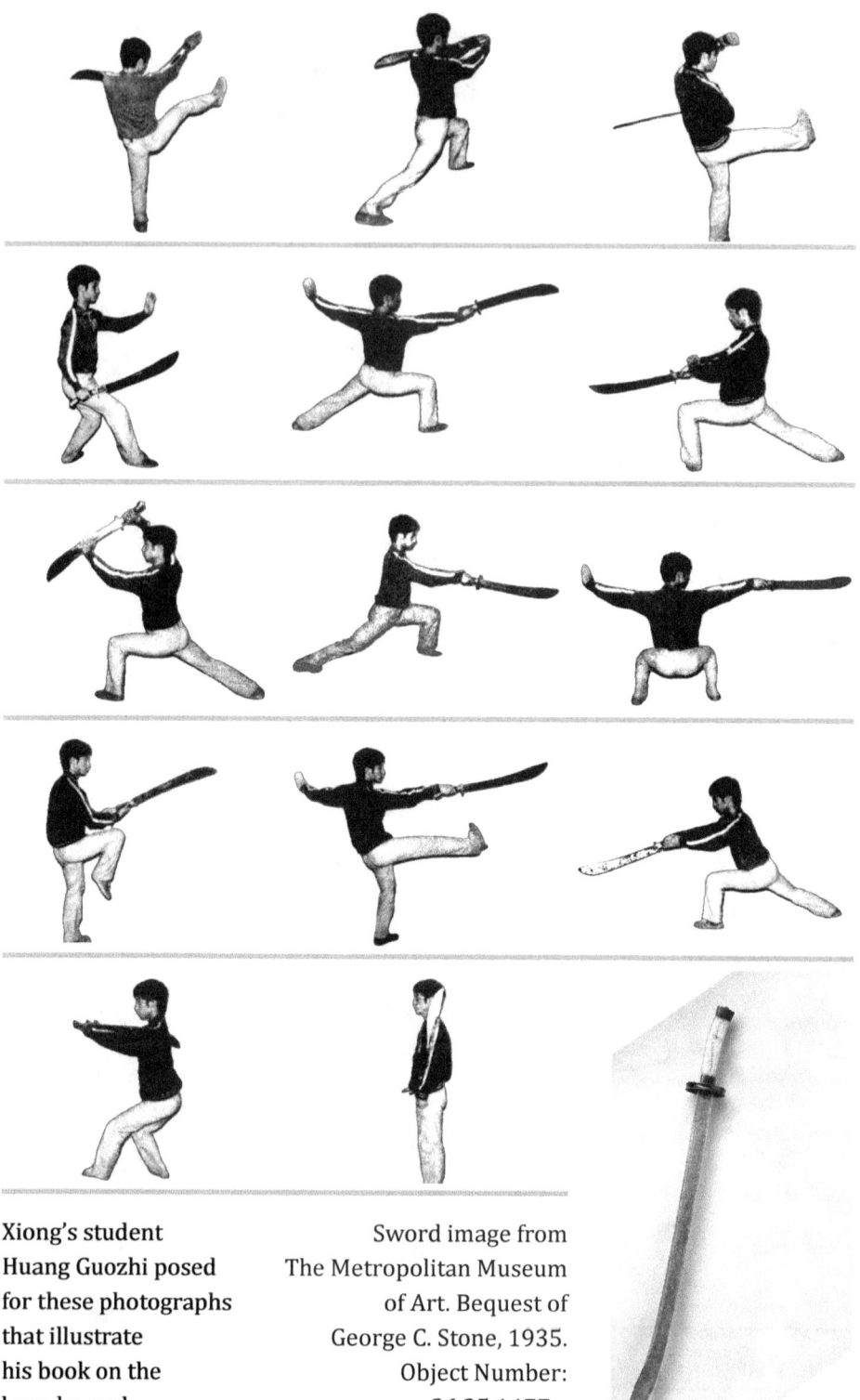

Xiong's student
Huang Guozhi posed
for these photographs
that illustrate
his book on the
broadsword.

Sword image from
The Metropolitan Museum
of Art. Bequest of
George C. Stone, 1935.
Object Number:
36.25.1477a.

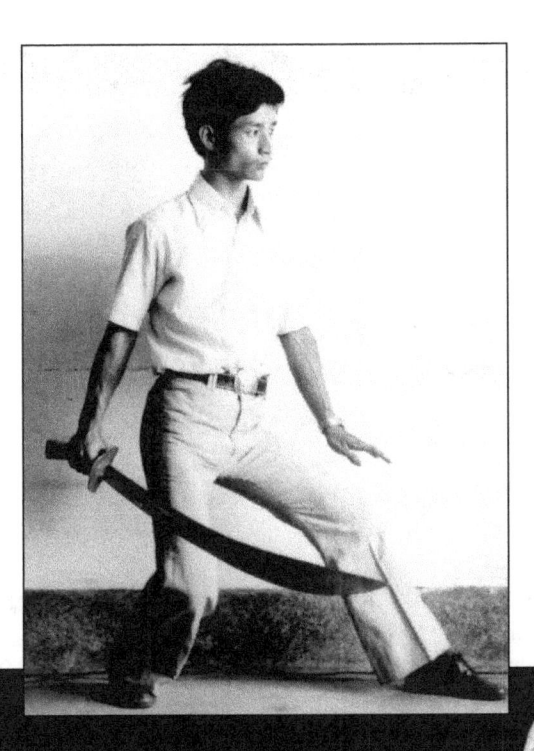

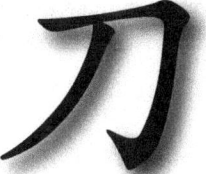

Left: Early photo of Huang Guozhi who appeared in Xiong Yanghe's book on the broadsword.

Below: A much more recent photo of Master Huang handling the broadsword.

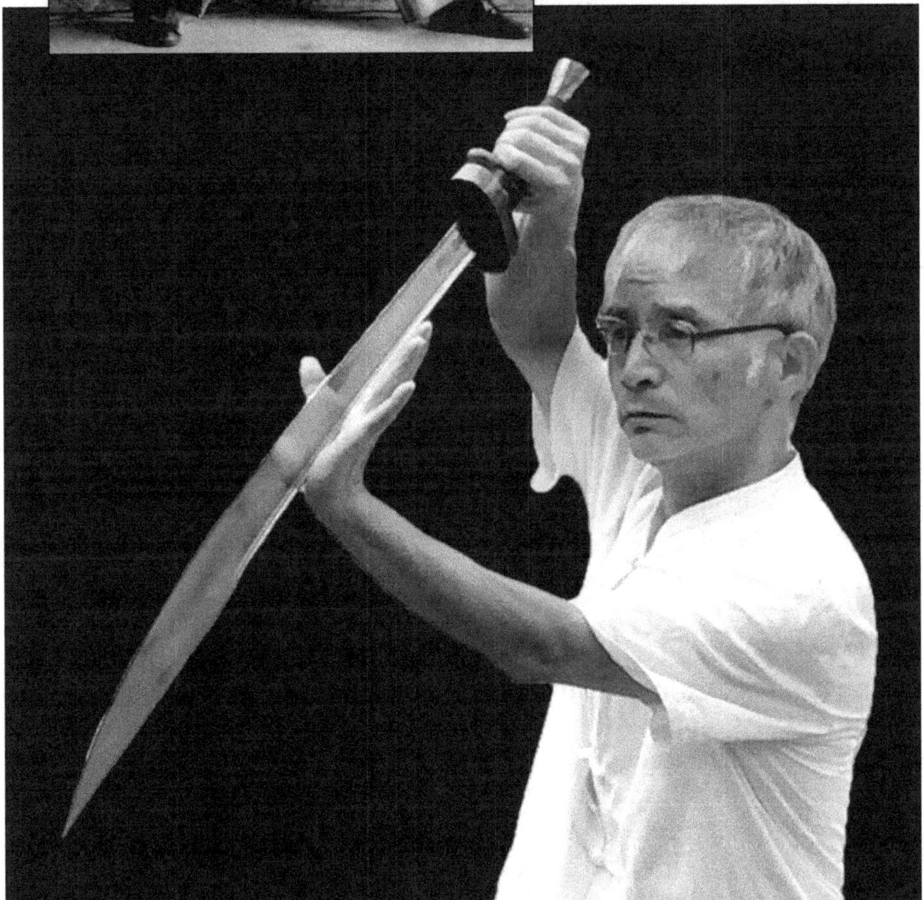

1) starting position   起勢
2) step forward to seven stars   上步七星
3) step back, turn left to seven stars   退步左轉七星
4) white crane spreads its wings   白鶴掠翅
5) turn, conceal the sword   轉身藏刀
6) split Mount Hua   力劈華山
7) step back, turn right and neutralize   退步右轉化
8) turn left, diagonal push sword to right   左鬆轉右斜推刀
9) turn right, upward intercept cut   右轉上截刀
10) turn and chop downward   轉身剁刀
11) turn left, dodge and neutralize, lift sword   左轉閃化撩刀
12) change step, turn, diagonal push cut   換步轉身斜推刀
13) evade with upward sword   閃避撩刀
14) step, turn, neutralize, left upward cut   換步轉身鬆化左撩刀
15) step forward, draw sword, turn draw up   上步招刀轉上招
16) turn, step forward, push boat with current   轉身上步順水推舟
17) turn, diagonal push cut   轉身斜推刀
18) turn, push boat with current   轉身順水推舟
19) turn, diagonal push cut   轉身斜推刀
20) step back, left scrape   退步左刮
21) step back, right scrape   退步右刮
22) step back, left scrape   退步左刮
23) step back, right scrape   退步右刮
24) turn, push boat with current   轉身順水推舟
25) turn, diagonal push cut   轉身斜推刀
26) turn, push boat with current   轉身順水推舟
27) turn, diagonal push cut   轉身斜推刀
28) step back, scrape left   退步左刮
29) step back, scrape right   退步右刮
30) step back, scrape left   退步左刮
31) step back, scrape right   退步右刮
32) turn, push boat with current   轉身順水推舟
33) jade lady threads at shuttle   玉女穿梭
34) turn, right fan strike   轉身右搧
35) jade lady threads at shuttle   玉女穿梭
36) turn, push boat with current   轉身順水推舟
37) turn left, right chop   左轉右劈刀
38) right dodge, chop downward   右閃剁刀
39) turn left, right chopcut   左轉右劈刀
40) closing of broadsword routine   收刀勢
41) ending posture   收刀歸原

1) starting position	起勢
2) step forward to seven stars	上步七星
3) step back, turn left to seven stars	退步左轉七星
4) white crane spreads its wings	白鶴掠翅
5) turn, conseal sword	轉身藏刀
6) turn, right chop	轉身右劈刀
7) step forward, upward thrust	進步撩刺刀
8) turn, chop with the flow	轉身順勢劈刀
9) change step, straight push cut	換步正推刀
10) withdraw, step forward, chop downward	撤換上步剁刀
11) turn, dodge to neutralize, horizonal pull	展轉閃化平拉
12) step back, right chop	退步右劈刀
13) neutralize, upward intercept, left scrape	鬆化上截左刮刀
14) step forward, right fan strike	上步右搧
15) step back, left scrape	退步左刮
16) step back, right scrape	退步右刮
17) step back, left scrape	退步左刮
18) step back, right scrape	退步右刮
19) push the boat with current	順水推舟
20) turn, diagonal push cut	轉身斜推刀
21) turn, push the boat with current	轉身順水推舟
22) turn, diagonal push cut	轉身斜推刀
23) step back, left scrape	退步左刮
24) step back, right scrape	退步右刮
25) step back, left scrape	退步左刮
26) step back, right scrape	退步右刮
27) turn, push the boat with current	轉身順水推舟
28) turn, diagonal push cut	轉身斜推刀
29) turn, push the boat with current	轉身順水推舟
30) turn, diagonal push cut	轉身斜推刀
31) step back, left scrape	退步左刮
32) turn left, right fan strike	左轉右搧
33) jade lady threads at shuttle	玉女穿梭
34) push the boat with current	順水推舟
35) jade lady threads at shuttle	玉女穿梭
36) turn, right chop	轉身右劈刀
37) right dodge, chop	右閃剁刀
38) turn left, right chop	左轉右劈刀
39) closing of broadsword routine	收刀勢
40) ending posture	收刀歸原

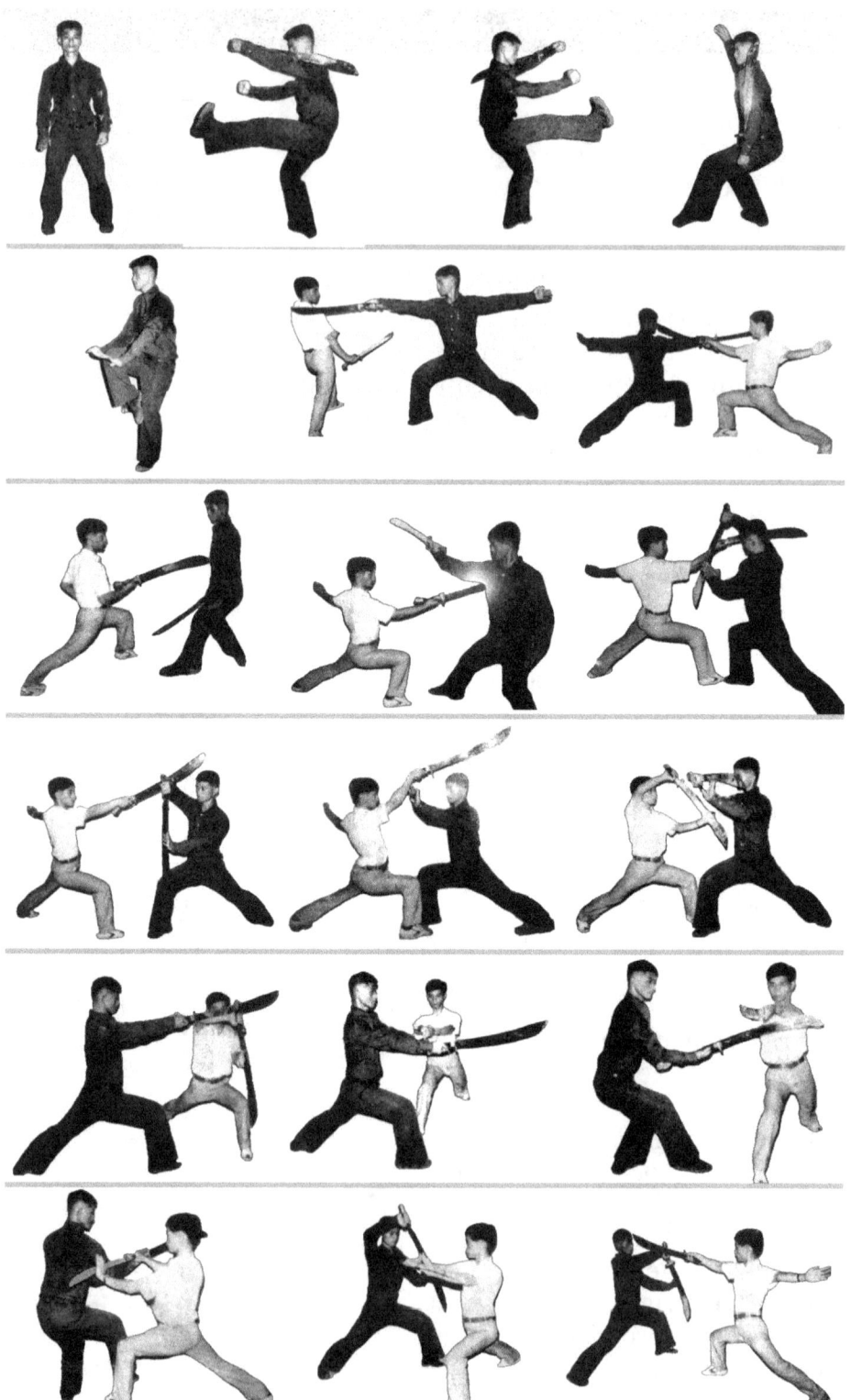

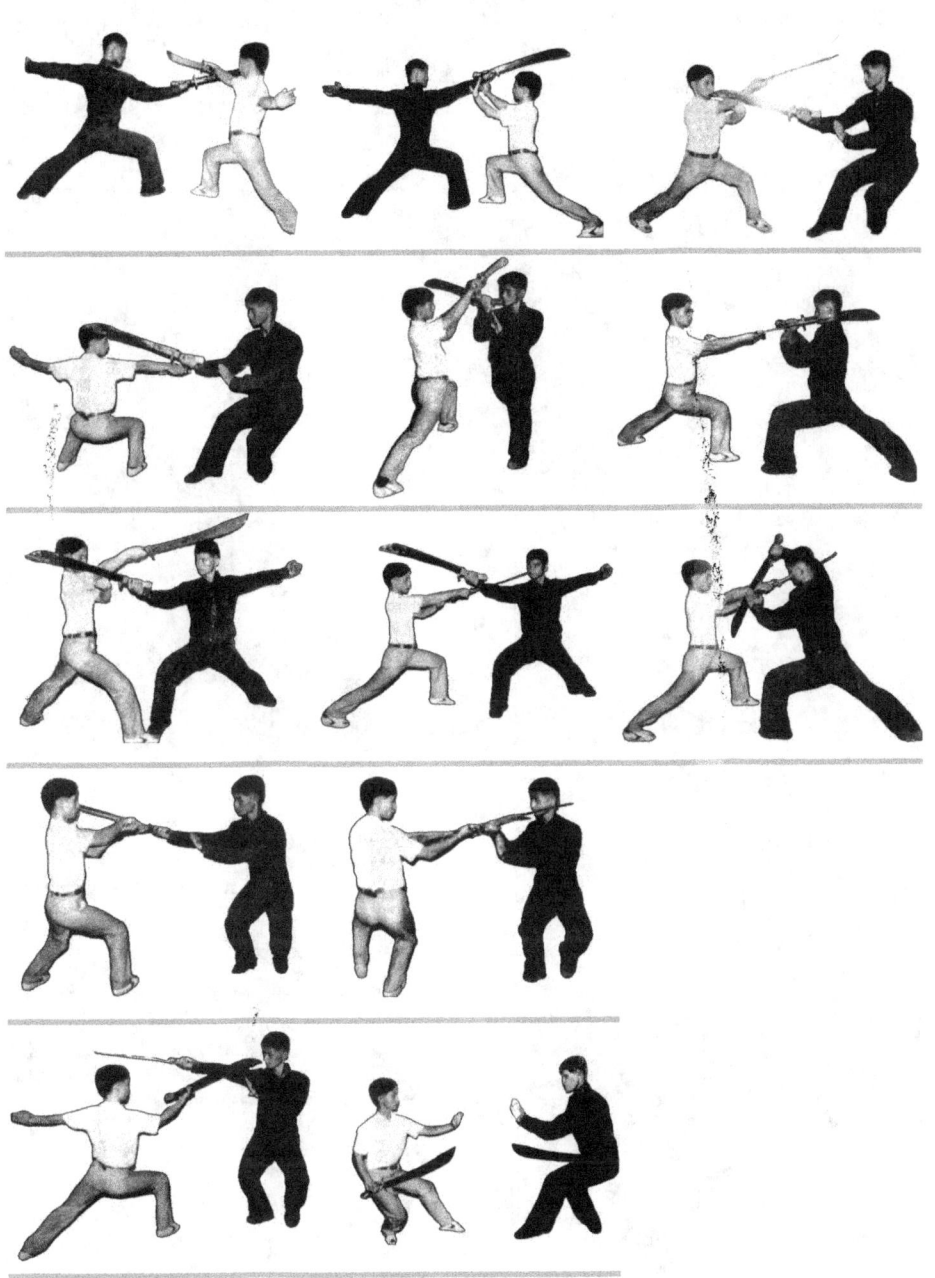

Xiong's students Huang Guozhi and Huang Qinglin posed for these photographs that illustrate his book on the broadsword.

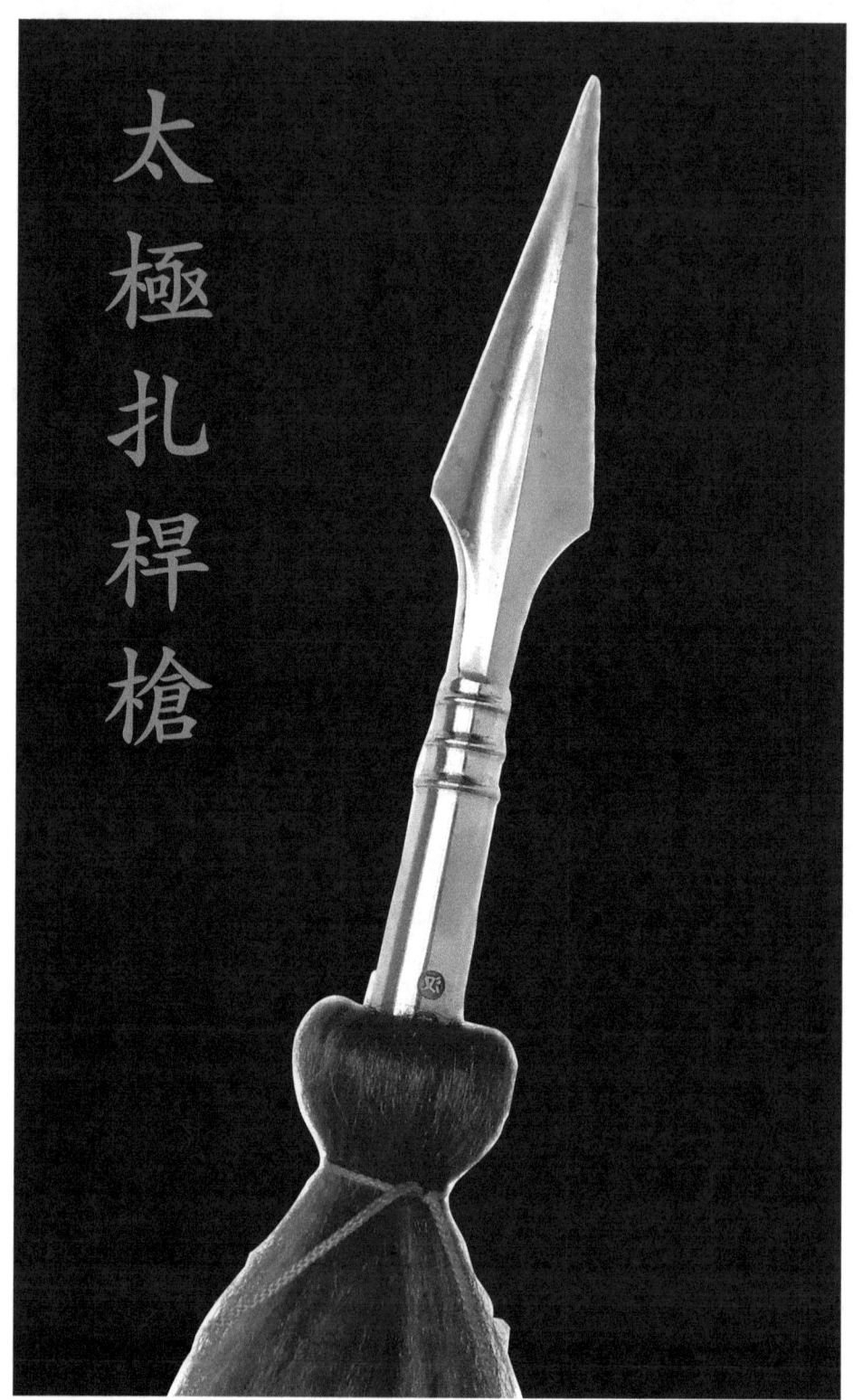

太極扎桿槍

‹ 8 ›

Taiji Staff /Spear Routines (solo/paired)

The *gun* or long staff has an advantage over many weapons in that it can keep opponents at a distance. This even includes animals! A long staff is considered the oldest weapon for good reasons, including aid in hunting or keeping fierce animals at bay.

The staff comes in different sizes and is often used in practical work. Especially in earlier days, it was placed over the shoulders for carrying water buckets and used for herding goats and sheep. Made of hard wax wood or rattan, the staff was a common item and proved useful in any type of combat. It is still found on farms and often in martial art schools.

Long weapons are a challenge for the martial artist because its length can make it difficult to control precisely. Some teachers talk about projecting the body's energy through the weapon. All weapons take time to master. One should eventually be able to move the end of the staff quickly to strike a tiny target, or a ping pong ball swinging through the air on a string. When you move a staff a few inches on the end closest to the body, the end furthest away can move two feet.

To use the staff well, the practitioner must always be aware where both ends are in space and how to use its length and ends in combative techniques.

In ancient times, an end of the staff would be burnt to make it slightly harder than normal. Add a sharp metal point to it and a formidable spear is made. The fighting techniques used for both staff and spear are very similar. Xiong's students would learn taiji staff and later study the Six Directions Flower Spear.

The overview of open-hand practices and weaponry as practiced in the Xiong system illustrate a richly complete system. Studies begin with the solo taiji routine and progresses to the open-hand duets and then to weaponry. Each practice trains the student in unique ways leading toward martial mastery.

1) beginning form　　　　　　　　　　　　　　　起勢

2) fixed stance, open-close, issue energy (1)　　　定步開合發(一)

3) fixed stance, open-close, issue energy (2)　　　定步開合發(二)

4) fixed stance, open-close, issue energy (3)　　　定步開合發(三)

5) fixed stance, open-close, issue energy (4)　　　定步開合發(四)

6) active step, open-close, issue energy (1)　　　活步開合發(一)

7) active step, open-close, issue energy (2)　　　活步開合發(二)

8) active step, open-close, issue energy (3)　　　活步開合發(三)

9) active step, open-close, issue energy (4)　　　活步開合發(四)

10) forward bow stance, thrust to chest (1)　　　前進弓步刺胸(一)

11) forward bow stance, thrust to leg (2)　　　前進弓步刺腿(二)

12) forward bow stance, thrust to shoulder (3)　　前進弓步刺肩 (三)

13) forward bow stance, thrust to throat (4)　　　前進弓步刺喉(四)

14) back horse stance, neutralize chest (1)　　　後退馬步化胸(一)

15) back horse stance, neutralize leg (2)　　　後退馬步化腿(二)

16) back horse stance, neutralize shoulder (3)　　後腿馬步化肩(三)

17) back horse stance, neutralize throat (4)　　　後退馬步化喉(四)

18) forward bow stance, thrust to chest (1)　　　前進弓步刺胸(一)

19) forward bow stance, thrust to leg (2)　　　前進弓步刺腿(二)

20) forward bow stance, thrust to shoulder (3)　　前進弓步刺肩(三)

21) forward bow stance, thrust to throat (4)　　　前進弓步刺喉(四)

22) back horse stance, neutralize chest (1)　　　後退馬步化胸(一)

23) back horse stance, neutralize leg (2)　　　後退馬步化腿(二)

24) back horse stance, neutralize shoulder (3)　　後退馬步化肩(三)

25) back horse stance, neutralize throat (4)　　　後退馬步化喉(四)

26) forward bow stance, thrust to leg (1)　　　前進弓步刺腿(一)

27) back one-leg stance, neutralize leg (2)　　　後退獨立步化腿(二)

28) forward bow stance, thrust to leg (3)　　　前進弓步刺腿(三)

29) back one-leg stance, neutralize leg (4)　　　後退獨立步化腿(四)

30) active step forward, thrust to leg (1)　　　活步前進刺腿(一)

31) active step backward, neutralize leg (2)　　　活步後退化腿 (二)

32) active step forward, thrust to leg (3)　　　活步前進刺腿(三)

33) active step backward, neutralize leg (4)　　　活步後退化腿(四)

34) active step forward, thrust to leg (1)　　　活步前進刺腿〔一〕

35) active step backward, hook step, neutralize leg (2)　　活步後退拐步化腿(二)

36) sidestep forward, bow stance, thrust to leg (3)	側步前進弓步刺腿(三)
37) sidestep forward, hook step, neutralize leg (4)	側步前進拐步化腿(四)
38) sidestep forward, bow stance, thrust to leg (5)	側步前進弓步刺腿(五)
39) **sidestep forward,** hook step, **neutralize leg (6)**	側步前進拐步化腿(六)
40) sidestep forward, bow stance, thrust to leg (7)	側步前進弓步刺腿(七)
41) sidestep forward, hook step, neutralize leg (8)	側步前進拐步化腿(八)
42) sidestep forward, bow stance, thrust to leg (9)	側步前進弓步刺腿(九)
43) sidestep forward, hook step, neutralize leg (10)	側步前進拐步化腿(十)
44) sidestep forward, bow stance, thrust to leg (11)	側步前進弓步刺腿(十一)
45) sidestep forward, hook step, neutralize leg (12)	側步前進拐步化腿(十二)
46) turn, advance bow stance, thrust to chest (1)	轉身前進弓步刺胸(一)
47) advance bow stance, thrust to leg (2)	前進弓步刺腿(二)
48) advance bow stance, thrust to chest (3)	前進弓步刺胸(三)
49) advance bow stance, thrust to leg (4)	前進弓步刺腿(四)
50) advance bow stance, thrust to chest (5)	前進弓步刺胸(五)
51) advance bow stance, thrust to leg (6)	前進弓步刺腿(六)
52) retreat horse stance, neutralize chest (1)	後退馬步化胸(一)
53) retreat horse stance neutralize leg (2)	後退馬步化腿(二)
54) retreat horse stance, neutralize chest (3)	後退馬步化胸(三)
55) retreat horse stance, neutralize leg (4)	後退馬步化腿(四)
56) retreat horse stance, neutralize chest (5)	後退馬步化胸(五)
57) retreat horse stance, neutralize leg (6)	後退馬步化腿(六)
58) advance bow stance, thrust to chest (1)	前進弓步刺胸(一)
59) advance bow stance, thrust to leg (2)	前進弓步刺腿(二)
60) advance bow stance, thrust to chest (3)	前進弓步刺胸(三)
61) advance bow stance, thrust to leg (4)	前進弓步刺腿(四)
62) advance bow stance, thrust to chest (5)	前進弓步刺胸(五)
63) advance bow stance, thrust to leg (6)	前進弓步刺腿(六)
64) retreat horse stance, neutralize chest (1)	後退馬步化胸(一)
65) retreat horse stance, neutralize leg (2)	後退馬步化腿(二)
66) retreat horse stance, neutralize chest (3)	後退馬步化胸(三)
67) retreat horse stance, neutralize leg (4)	後退馬步化腿(四)
68) retreat horse stance, neutralize chest (5)	後退馬步化胸(五)
69) retreat horse stance, neutralize leg (6)	後退馬步化腿(六)
70) pivot, bow stance, lift and block overhead	原地轉身弓步上架
71) ending, return to the original posture	收勢歸原

Starting position (A position)

1) beginning
2) fixed step, open-close, issue energy (1)
3) fixed step, open-close, issue energy (2)
4) fixed step, open-close, issue energy (3)
5) fixed step, open-close, issue energy (4)
6) active step, open-close, issue energy (1)
7) active step, open-close, issue energy (2)
8) active step, open-close, issue energy (3)
9) active step, open-close, issue energy (4)
10) forward bow stance, thrust to chest (1)
11) forward bow stance, thrust to leg (2)
12) forward bow stance, thrust to shoulder (3)
13) forward bow stance, thrust to throat (4)
14) back horse stance, neutralize chest (1)
15) back horse stance, neutralize leg (2)
16) back horse stance, neutralize shoulder (3)
17) back horse stance, neutralize throat (4)
18) forward bow stance, thrust to chest (1)
19) forward bow stance, thrust to leg (2)
20) forward bow stance, thrust to shoulder (3)
21) forward bow stance, thrust to throat (4)
22) back horse stance, neutralize chest (1)
23) back horse stance, neutralize leg (2)
24) back horse stance, neutralize shoulder (3)
25) back horse stance, neutralize throat (4)
26) forward bow stance, thrust to leg (1)
27) back single-leg stance, neutralize leg (2)
28) forward bow stance, thrust to leg (3)
29) back single-leg stance, neutralize leg (4)
30) active forward bow stance, thrust to leg (1)
31) active step, neutralize leg (2)
32) active step forward, thrust to leg (3)
33) active step back, neautral leg (4)
34) active step forward, thrust to leg (1)
35) active step back, turn, neutralize leg (2)
36) sidestep forward, bow stance, thrust to leg (3)
37) sidestep forward, turning stance, neutralize leg (4)
38) sidestep forward, bow stance, thrust to leg (5)
39) sidestep forward, turning stance, neutralize leg (6)

40) sidestep forward, bow stance, thrust to leg (7)
41) sidestep forward, turning stance, neutralize leg (8)
42) sidestep forward, bow stance, thrust to leg (9)
43) sidestep forward, turning stance, neutralize leg (10)
44) sidestep forward, bow stance, thrust to leg (11)
45) sidestep forward, turning stance, neutralize leg (12)
46) turn, advance with bow stance, thrust to chest (1)
47) advance with bow stance, thrust to leg (2)
48) advance with bow stance, thrust to chest (3)
49) advance with bow stance, thrust to leg (4)
50) advance with bow stance, thrust to chest (5)
51) advance with bow stance, thrust to leg (6)
52) retreating horse stance, neutralize chest (1)
53) retreating horse stance, neutralize leg (2)
54) retreating horse stance, neutralize chest (3)
55) retreating horse stance, neutralize leg (4)
56) retreating horse stance, neutralize chest (5)
57) retreating horse stance, neutralize leg (6)
58) advance with bow stance, thrust to chest (1)
59) advance with bow stance, thrust to leg (2)
60) advance with bow stance, thrust to chest (3)
61) advance with bow stance, thrust to leg (4)
62) advance with bow stance, thrust to chest (5)
63) advance with bow stance, thrust to leg (6)
64) retreating horse stance, neutralize chest (1)
65) retreating horse stance, neutralize leg (2)
66) retreating horse stance, neutralize chest (3)
67) retreating horse stance, neutralize leg (4)
68) retreating horse stance, neutralize chest (5)
69) retreating horse stance, neutralize leg (6)
70) turn in place, bow stance, upward thrust
71) concluding form, return to the original posture

Starting position (B position)

1) beginning
2) fixed stance, open-close, issue energy (1)
3) fixed stance, open-close, issue energy (2)
4) fixed stance, open-close, issue energy (3)
5) fixed stance, open-close, issue energy (4)
6) active step, open-close, issue energy (1)
7) active step, open-close, issue energy (2)
8) active step, open-close, issue energy (3)
9) active step, open-close, issue energy (4)
10) back horse stance, neutralize chest (1)
11) back horse stance, neutralize leg (2)
12) back horse stance, neutralize shoulder (3)
13) back horse stance, neutralize throat (4)
14) step forward bow stance, thrust to chest (1)
15) step forward bow stance, thrust to leg (2)
16) step forward bow stance, thrust to shoulder (3)
17) step forward bow stance, thrust to throat (4)
18) back horse stance, neutralize chest (1)
19) back horse stance, neutralize leg (2)
20) back horse stance, neutralize shoulders (3)
21) back horse stance, neutralize throat (4)
22) step forward bow stance, thrust to chest (1)
23) step forward bow stance, thrust to leg (2)
24) step forward bow stance, thrust to shoulder (3)
25) step forward bow stance, thrust to throat (4)
26) step back one-leg stance, neutralize leg (1)
27) step forward bow stance, thrust to leg (2)
28) step back one-leg stance, neutralize leg (3)
29) step forward bow stance, thrust to leg (4)
30) active step back, neutralize leg (1)
31) active step forward, thrust to leg (2)
32) active step back, neutralize leg (3)
33) active step forward, thrust to leg (4)
34) active step back with hook step, neutralize leg (1)
35) sidestep forward bow stance, thrust to leg (2)
36) sidestep forward with hook step, neutralize leg (3)
37) sidestep forward bow stance, thrust to leg (4)
38) sidestep forward with hook step, neutralize leg (5)
39) sidestep forward bow stance, thrust to leg (6)
40) sidestep forward, with hook step, neutralize leg (7)
41) sidestep forward bow stance, thrust to kick (8)

42) sidestep forward with hook step, neutralize leg (9)
43) sidestep forward bow stance, thrust to leg (10)
44) sidestep forward with hook step, neutralize leg (11)
45) sidestep forward bow stance, thrust to leg (12)
46) back horse stance, neutralize chest (1)
47) back horse stance, neutralize leg (2)
48) back horse stance, neutralize chest (3)
49) back horse stance, neutralize leg (4)
50) back horse stance, neutralize chest (5)
51) back horse stance, neutralize leg (6)
52) forward bow stance, thrust to chest (1)
53) forward bow stance, thrust to leg (2)
54) forward bow stance, thrust to chest (3)
55) forward bow stance, thrust to leg (4)
56) forward bow stance, thrust to chest (5)
57) forward bow stance, thrust to leg (6)
58) back horse stance, neutralize chest (1)
59) back horse stance, neutralize leg (2)
60) back horse stance, neutralize chest (3)
61) back horse stance, neutralize leg (4)
62) back horse stance, neutralize chest (5)
63) back horse stance, neutralize leg (6)
64) forward bow stance, thrust to chest (1)
65) forward bow stance, thrust to leg (2)
66) forward bow stance, thrust to chest (3)
67) forward bow stance, lunge (4)
68) forward bow stance, thrust to chest (5)
69) forward bow stance, thrust to leg (6)
70) turn in place, bow stance, raise and block overhead
71) closing form, return to the original posture

上手(甲勢)

1) 起勢
2) 定步開合發(一)
3) 定步開合發(二)
4) 定步開合發(三)
5) 定步開合發(四)
6) 活步開合發(一)
7) 活步開合發(二)
8) 活步開合發(三)
9) 活步開合發(四)
10) 前進弓步刺胸(一)
11) 前進弓步刺腿(二)
12) 前進弓步刺肩(三)
13) 前進弓步刺喉(四)
14) 後退馬步化胸(-)
15) 後退馬步化腿(二)
16) 後退馬步化肩(三)
17) 後退馬步化喉(四)
18) 前進弓步刺胸(一)
19) 前進弓步刺腿(二)
20) 前進弓步刺肩(三)
21) 前進弓步刺喉(四)
22) 後退馬步化胸(一)
23) 後退馬步化腿(二)
24) 後退馬步化肩(三)
25) 後退馬步化喉(四)
26) 前進弓步刺腿(一)
27) 後退獨立步化腿(二)
28) 前進弓步刺腿(三)
29) 後退獨立步化腿(四)
30) 活步前進刺腿(一)
31) 活步後退化腿(二)
32) 活步前進刺腿(三)
33) 活步後退化腿(四)
34) 活步前進刺腿(一)
35) 活步後退拐步化腿(二)
36) 側步前進弓步刺腿(三)

下手(乙勢)

1) 起勢
2) 定步開合發(一)
3) 定步開合發(二)
4) 定步開合發(三)
5) 定步開合發(四)
6) 活步開合發(一)
7) 活步開合發(二)
8) 活步開合發(三)
9) 活步開合發(四)
10) 後退馬步化胸(一)
11) 後退馬步化腿(二)
12) 後退馬步化肩 (三)
13) 後退馬步化喉(四)
14) 前進弓步刺胸(一)
15) 前進弓步刺腿(二)
16) 前進弓步刺肩(三)
17) 前進弓步刺喉(四)
18) 後退馬步化胸(一)
19) 後退馬步化腿(二)
20) 後退馬步化肩(三)
21) 後退馬步化喉(四)
22) 前進弓步刺胸(一)
23) 前進弓步刺腿(二)
24) 前進弓步刺肩(三)
25) 前進弓步刺喉(四)
26) 後退獨立步化腿(一)
27) 前進弓步刺腿(二)
28) 後退獨立步化腿(三)
29) 前進弓步刺腿(四)
30) 活步後退化腿(一)
31) 活步前進刺腿(二)
32) 活步後退化腿(三)
33) 活步前進刺腿(四)
34) 活步後退拐步化腿(一)
35) 側步前進弓步刺腿(二)
36) 側步前進拐步化腿(三)

37) 側步前進拐步化腿(四)
38) 側步前進弓步刺腿(五)
39) 側步前進拐步化腿(六)
40) 側步前進弓步刺腿(七)
41) 側步前進拐步化腿(八)
42) 側步前進弓步刺腿(九)
43) 側步前進拐步化腿(十)
44) 側步前進弓步刺腿(十一)
45) 側步前進拐步化腿(十二)
46) 轉身前進弓步刺胸(一)
47) 前進弓步刺腿(二)
48) 前進弓步刺胸(三)
49) 前進弓步刺腿(四)
50) 前進弓步刺胸(五)
51) 前進弓步刺腿(六)
52) 後退馬步化胸(一)
53) 後退馬步化腿(二)
54) 後退馬步化胸(三)
55) 後退馬步化腿(四)
56) 後退馬步化胸(五)
57) 後退馬步化腿(六)
58) 前進弓步刺胸(一)
59) 前進弓步刺腿(二)
60) 前進弓步刺胸(三)
61) 前進弓步刺腿(四)
62) 前進弓步刺胸(五)
63) 前進弓步刺腿(六)
64) 後退馬步化胸(一)
65) 後退馬步化腿(二)
66) 後退馬步化胸(三)
67) 後退馬步化腿(四)
68) 後退馬步化胸(五)
69) 後退馬步化腿(六)
70) 原地轉身弓步上架
71) 收勢歸原

37) 側步前進弓步刺腿(四)
38) 側步前進拐步化腿(五)
39) 側步前進弓步刺腿(六)
40) 側步前進拐步化腿(七)
41) 側步前進弓步刺腿(八)
42) 側步前進拐步化腿(九)
43) 側步前進弓步刺腿(十)
44) 側步前進拐步化腿(十一)
45) 側步前進弓步刺腿(十二)
46) 後退馬步化胸(一)
47) 後退馬步化腿(二)
48) 後退馬步化胸(三)
49) 後退馬步化腿(四)
50) 後退馬步化胸(五)
51) 後退馬步化腿(六)
52) 前進弓步刺胸(一)
53) 前進弓步刺腿(二)
54) 前進弓步刺胸(三)
55) 前進弓步刺腿(四)
56) 前進弓步刺胸(五)
57) 前進弓步刺腿(六)
58) 後退馬步化胸(一)
59) 後退馬步化腿(二)
60) 後退馬步化胸(三)
61) 後退馬步化腿(四)
62) 後退馬步化胸(五)
63) 後退馬步化腿(六)
64) 前進弓步刺胸(一)
65) 前進弓步刺腿(二)
66) 前進弓步刺胸(三)
67) 前進弓步刺腿(四)
68) 前進弓步刺胸(五)
69) 前進弓步刺腿(六)
70) 原地轉身弓步上架
71) 收勢歸原

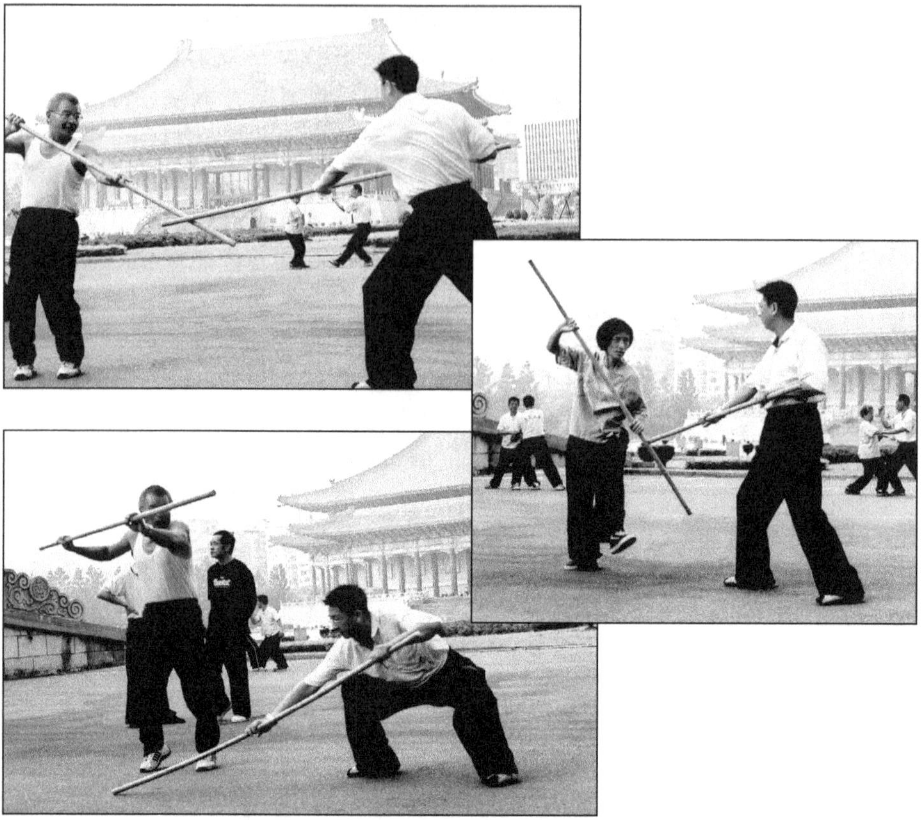

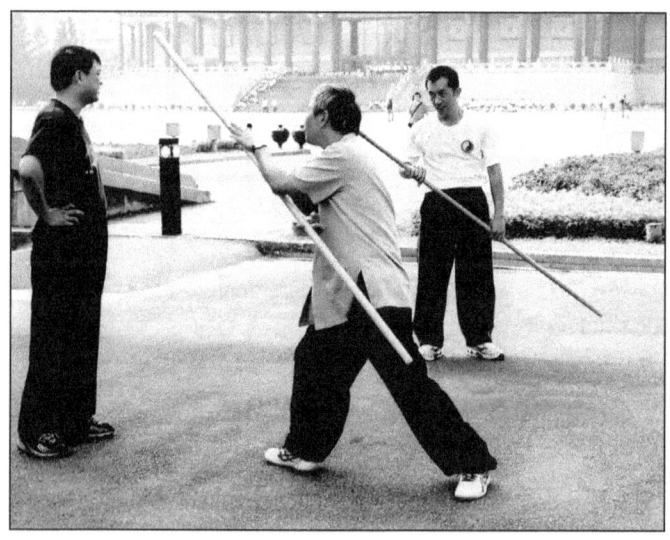

Above right: Master Lin Jianhong (right center) studied primarily under Guo Tingxian (1925-2002). Here in Taipei he is instructing some students in long staff.

◀ 9 ▶

Bonus of the Five Animal Frolics

"Lions, and tigers, and bears . . . Oh my!" — This famous quote from the 1939 movie classic *The Wizard of Oz* is a very fitting response when one first sees the Five Animal Frolics (*wuqinxi*) being practiced in Taiwan. This system of exercise—said to be the earliest form of medical qigong—is based primarily on the movements of five animals: the ape, bear, crane, deer, and tiger. A famed Chinese physician, Hua Tuo, is credited for developing these exercises around 200 C.E. by observing animals and applying his knowledge of anatomy, acupuncture, moxibustion, and medicine.

There is some information available in Western countries regarding Hua Tuo and the Five Animal Frolics, primarily about the exercise as practiced on mainland China. This presentation focuses on the exercises as they developed in Taiwan. We will invistigate the leading figures responsible for bringing the practices to Taiwan and discover how and why the Five Animal Frolics are beneficial as a method of rehabilitation and, more importantly, as exercises for nurturing health and preventing disease and infirmity.

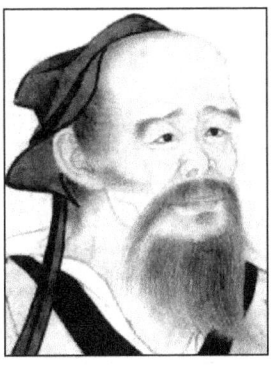

Dr. Hua Tuo

Bearers of Gifts

Following the civil war on mainland China (1927-1950), approximately two million people fled the Communist takeover and migrated to the island of Taiwan. Many were military men, including some notable martial art masters. One of these stellar figures was Zhang Jingying (張鏡影 1899-1980). During the Second Sino-Japanese War (1937-1945), Zhang knew an official who was shot in the leg and doctors felt it best to amputate due to the wound's severity. Luckily a Daoist was called in to see if a traditional method of healing would work. It did, inspiring Zhang to study healing methods—including the Five Animal Frolics—with Daoists of Qingcheng Mountain in Sichuan Province. Zhang became a 77th generation master in this system and the first person to teach Hua Tuo's art in Taiwan.

Over the centuries, the Five Animal Frolics have been passed on over generations by secret transmission. On the mainland, the Communists had suppressed old traditional practices, even executing noted martial art and qigong masters. In Taiwan, there was great concern for preserving the ancient traditions, especially the health-related modalities. Zhang Jigying started teaching the Five Animals to a small group at the legislative Yuan (parliament) in 1956. More than eighty people began studying the original 125-movement version. Most could not master this lengthy series of subtle exercises. Only two were successful. Zhang Jingying made a rule that the number of apprentices must not exceed five. His talented disciples included Yu Zhongyu, Wang Huazhong, Hu Guofan, Deng Fuyu, and Guo Tingxian: representing the 78th generation representatives of the art. Most of the men who were trained by him were martial artists.

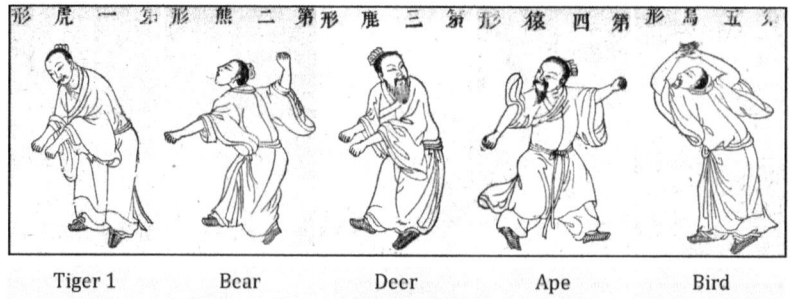

Five Animal images from *The Cinnabar Book of Longevity*.
Courtesy of the Wellcome Collection.

Animal Frolic	Element	Yin Organ	Yang Organ	Emotion
Ape	Earth	Spleen	Stomach	Worry
Bear	Wood	Liver	Gall Bladder	Anger
Bird	Fire	Heart	Small Intestines	Joy
Deer	Water	Kidneys	Bladder	Fear
Tiger	Metal	Lung	Large Intestines	Sadness

One of the five disciples under Mr. Zhang Jingying was Mr. Guo Tingxian (1925-2002). It is to his credit that the Five Animals popularity spread throughout Taiwan. He and his disciples started an institute to research and teach his system. Mr. Guo devised abridged routines based on Zhang Jingying's original version, making it easier to promote.[1]

Guo had also studied with a few martial art masters. In 1956 he became a disciple of Master Xiong Yanghe (1889-1981). Guo had Xiong's support and encouragement for teaching the Five Animal Frolics. Many of Xiong's students learned from Guo. Branches of Guo's institute later opened in other locations.

Another close friend of Master Xiong was Mr. Li Qinghan, who also studied the Five Animals system under Zhang Jingying. Li taught some of Xiong's students too. Li taught four versions: (1) one following the original by Zhang Jingying, (2) another with some of the repeated movements removed, (3) a concise routine, and (4) a simplified version.

Blending Exercise with Medical Theory

In Hua Tuo's time, Chinese traditional medicine had already been well established in theory and practice. The foundation of Chinese medical practice is based on an understanding of the body and its relation to the movement of inner energies. Thus, the Chinese practical application of the Five Elements (*wuxing*) and energetic meridians were likewise employed in design of the Five Animal Frolics practice. The Five Elements are symbolic of the five organs of the body. All the animals move differently and so each human replication effects the body in different ways. When the animal gestures are imitated by a human, the movements stimulate corresponding inner organs. Some movements stimulate yin organs and other movements stimulate yang organs (*zhang/fu*).

Practice Method: Become the Animal

The exercises are performed by physically imitating the movements of each animal. Some may even imitate how they breathe, move spontaneously, or emit sounds that correspond to a particular animal. Most masters teach standard forms of movements although schools have their variations. It is the same phenomenon seen in taijiquan with its varieties, manifested according to the skills and insights of the teacher.

The peculiarities of each animal movement can be understood by their unique effect on the body: loosening joints, stretching specific tendons and muscle groups, pressing on selected organs, and pumping blood, oxygen, and qi through passages to invigorate the system. With the intestines massaged by movement, digestion is improved. Hand gestures activate energy flow as does the touching of acupoints and tracing meridians as part of specific movements. Gulping down breath effects respiration. Gentle bending and extending of the limbs make the spine more flexible.

University studies in Shanghai show that practitioners demonstrated improvements in immunity function. An article in the *Journal of Physical Therapy Science* states that the Animal Frolic exercises exemplify a method of reducing lower back pain. In all, the dynamic Animal Frolics certainly put one's body through postures on par with those found in static yoga. Such an array of movement has great effect on all the bodily systems.

The mental aspect involved in these exercises plays a large role in gaining results. A practitioner utilizes relaxation and "intention" to guide qi to pass through the seventy-two major joints as the movements facilitate the energy flow. As the Animal Frolics are usually taught within a traditional teacher-disciple relationship, a knowledgeable teacher may provide valuable instruction that goes beyond common practice.

Some practitioners try to absorb character traits of the individual animals, be it a deer's grace, a tiger's dignity, a bear's strength, a bird's freedom, or an ape's liveliness. The actual effect here is mostly subconscious. The degree varies according to everyone's capacity to manifest the animal characteristics in their personalities.

As in taijiquan, the Five Animal exercises calm the inside with slow movements, quieting the nerves and soothing the breath. Unlike taijiquan, however, the prime goal of the Animal Frolics is different. Taiji was originally designed for combat where the extension of movements is purposefully not executed to an extreme. For example, an overly outstretched arm or leg can easily be broken by an attacker. Also, a body that is twisted to an extreme can be easily toppled. The great value of the Animal Frolics is that they were designed not for self-defense, but for nurturing health. The animal movements go to extremes by stretching and pulling the body in a variety of positions, loosening the joints, and lengthening the muscles (the very definition of *daoyin*).

Variants on the Theme

Although Hua Tuo is credited for creating the Five Animal Frolics, we cannot know for sure exactly how they looked originally. There are some ancient illustrations that have survived the centuries that serve as a reference. An early publication containing clear wood-block images is *The Cinnabar Book of Longevity* written by Gong Juzhong during the Ming Dynasty (1368-1644).

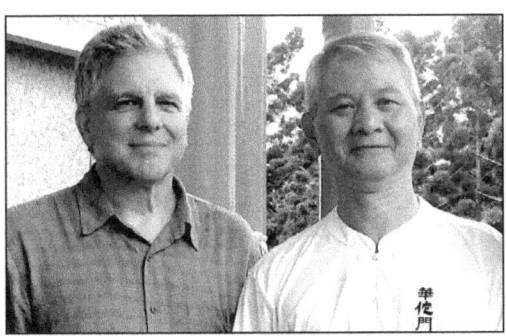

In Chiang Kai-shek Memorial Park, Taipei,
where the author enjoyed practicing the
Animal Frolics with Lin Jianhong.

A version being taught by Lin Jianhong—a disciple of Guo Ting-xian and a 79th generation representative of the Hua Tuo Five Animals Frolics—contains a total of 84 movements in eight sections. It is a complex routine of successive movements, requiring that the practitioner move slowly with deep relaxation. For overall health, the full 84-movement sequence can be performed. If this seems overwhelming, only one section or a few sections can be done in repetition. From the health perspective, a practitioner can select specific animal movements for specific needs. It would be best to seek advice from someone who is very familiar with the Frolics for such specifics.

Hua Tuo's Five Animal Frolics represent a gem of Chinese physical culture, packaged in a joyful exercise modeled on playful animals. Learning is fun with many benefits to give incentive for the practitioner to train regularly. Plus, there is no need to fear "lions, and tigers, and bears!"

Sample Movements to Practice

In the following sequence, the author practices four movements from the 84-movement Five Animal Frolics routine. As in the Yang-style solo form of taijiquan, each movement flows from one into the next. The practitioner should be very relaxed, moving slowly through the sequence.

1-2) Tiger Pounces Right
From the previous movement called Ape Lifts Arms, the tiger scrapes downward with its paws as its body shifts and sinks back into the left leg.

3-6) Crane Extends Wing to the Left
While the waist is turning left, the arms are led toward the left side. As one starts shifting right, the left arm reaches far left while the right hand flows to rest on the left side. The waist continues turning right with the left arm extending straight to the side, following an arch as it moves upward and to the right side of the body—as a crane extends its wing.

7-9) Bear Passes to the Left
As the left arm lowers to shoulder height (#7), it bends slightly at the elbow, and the body starts shifting left. A relaxed back and spine allow the elbow to reach its furthest point behind the left side.

10-15 Deer Rubs Side of the Neck
At this point, one lowers the torso toward the left side, allowing the right hand to meet under the left, and moving the torso further downward toward to the left knee. (Note: the forearm appears to turn downward, but it is following the angle of the turning spine). As the torso curves toward the right knee, the right arm extends as the left hand slides naturally to right forearm with the index finger stopping at the Lung 7 (LU 7) acupoint. As the torso rises (#13), the spine is rotated at an angle, causing the right elbow to rotate left while the hand moves right—as a deer would rub its neck (#14). From this angle, the practitioner starts to flow into the next movement (crane extends right wing).

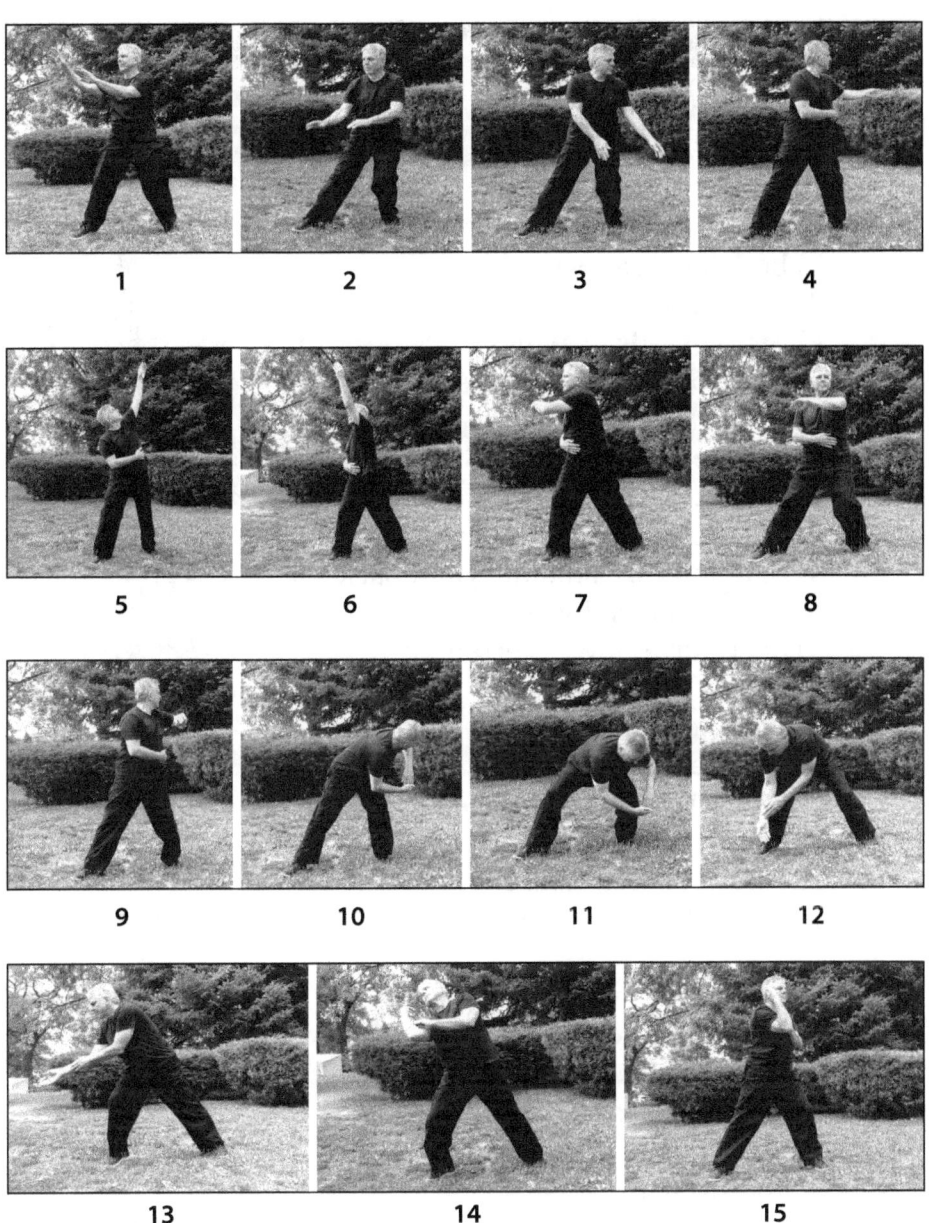

Trying the above sequence hopefully will give you an experience how the Five Animal Frolics can benefit practitioners. Keep in mind that eighty more movements are necessary for the full effect! Other movements require foot movements, kicking, being on one leg, squatting, relaxing the joints and muscles, and a loose twisting of all the vertebrae.

Technical photographs by Meade Martin. All other photos except Hua Tuo are courtesy of M. DeMarco and Lin Jianhong.

Guo Tingxian's Version

Sec. 1: Preparation   第一節預備功
1) standing deer gazing into distance   鹿站遠眺
2) bear bends at waist   熊俯身腰
3) white ape offers fruit   白猿獻果
4) bird spreads its wings   鳥展雙翅
5) tiger loosens its shoulders and back   虎鬆肩背

Sec 2: Red Phoenix Facing the Sun   第二節丹鳳朝陽
1) ape lifts arms   猿臂正舉
2) white crane expands chest   白鶴張胸
3) tiger loosens shoulders and back   虎鬆肩背
4) bear ascends tiptoe   熊攀足尖
5) deer moves lower vertebrae   鹿運脊尾
6) ape lifts right arm   猿臂右舉
7) tiger pounces right   右虎撲式
8) crane extends left wing   鶴展左翅
9) bear circulates energy left   左運熊經
10) right hand rubs deer's neck   右揉鹿頸
11) crane spreads right wing   鶴展右翅
12) beat the side, strengthen liver   拍脅強肝

Sec. 3: Golden Rooster Hatching Eggs   第三節金雞孵蛋
1) tiger squats down   虎踞沉坐
2) ape stretches right arm   猿舒右臂
3) ape stretches left arm   猿舒左臂
4) bear squats, embraces right   熊蹲右抱
5) ape stretches left arm   猿舒左臂
6) golden rooster stands on one leg   金雞獨立
7) crane fans right wing   鶴搧右翅
8) deer running, flees right   右旋鹿奔
9) raging tiger searches mountain   怒虎搜山
10) ape stretches right arm   猿舒右臂
11) bear squats, embraces left   熊蹲左抱
12) white crane embraces chest   白鶴抱胸
13) clever ape picks fruit   靈猿摘果

90

Sec. 4: Mythical Bird Spreads Wings 　　第四節大鵬展翅
    1) tiger turns right to sit 　　虎旋右坐
    2) ape dodges by turning left 　　猿閃左盤
    3) right, golden rooster stands 　　右金雞獨立靈猿
    4) clever ape points to the sun 　　指日
    5) deer looks back 　　鹿仰回顧
    6) bear moves waist and hips 　　熊運腰胯
    7) golden rooster stands, left 　　左金雞獨立
    8) right, rhinoceros gazes at full moon 　　右犀牛望月
    9) left, rhinoceros gazes at full moon 　　左犀牛望月
    10) white crane embracing the elixir 　　白鶴抱丹
    11) ape manages the triple burner 　　猿理三蕉
    12) bear wiggles the viscera 　　熊蠕臟腑
    13) fierce tiger goes down the mountain 　　猛虎下山
    14) deer stretches to the right 　　鹿引右盤
    15) white crane, twist step 　　白鶴拗步
    16) bear leans, tiger squats 　　熊靠虎踞

Sec. 5: Peacock Opens Its Shield 　　第五節孔雀開屏
    1) ape extends right arm backward 　　右猿臂反伸
    2) bear moves shoulders and hips 　　熊運肩胯
    3) tiger claw seizing attack 　　虎掌抓撲
    4) white crane expands chest 　　白鶴張胸
    5) staring owl 　　鴟眼顧盼
    6) white python turns its body 　　白蟒翻身
    7) black bear climbs downward 　　黑熊倒攀
    8) ape extends its arm backward, left 　　左猿臂反伸
    9) clever ape picks fruit 　　靈猿摘果

Sec. 6: Magpie Ascends to a Branch 　　第六節喜鵲登枝
    1) tiger pounces, deer runs 　　虎撲鹿奔
    2) crane stands on one leg, right 　　右鶴獨立
    3) deer butts and kicks, left 　　左鹿骶蹬蹄
    4) bear sits down cross-legged, left 　　熊左盤坐
    5) crane stands on one leg, left 　　左鶴獨立
    6) deer butts and kicks, right 　　右鹿骶蹬蹄
    7) ape hits tiger, right 　　猿右打虎
    8) bear resists, leans left 　　熊左抗靠
    9) bird stretchs, twisting-step 　　拗步鳥伸
    10) tiger pounces, counter strikes 　　虎撲反捶

11) deer turns, coiling left　　　　鹿旋左盤
12) bear resists, leans right　　　熊右抗靠
13) bear resists, leans left　　　　熊左抗靠
14) ape dodges, deer leads　　　　猿閃鹿引
15) tiger turns right to sit　　　　右轉虎坐
16) tiger claws foreward, backward　前後虎掌
17) white crane flying　　　　　　白鶴飛翔

Sec. 7: Red Phoenix Greets the Sun　　第七節丹鳳朝陽
1) ape lifts left arm　　　　　　　猿臂左舉
2) grabbing tiger takes a seat　　虎抓下坐
3) crane spreads left wing　　　　鶴展左翅
4) bear circulates energy right　　右運熊經
5) left hand rubs deer's neck　　　左揉鹿頸
6) ape lifts left arm　　　　　　　猿臂左舉
7) grabbing tiger takes a seat　　虎抓下坐
8) ape lifts right arm　　　　　　猿臂右舉
9) turn around, collect power　　轉身收勢

Sec. 8: Receiving Benefits　　　　第八節收功
1) rotate and rub the deer's neck　旋揉鹿頸
2) bear sways, owl glances around　熊晃鴟顧
3) immortal fox bows to the moon　仙狐拜月

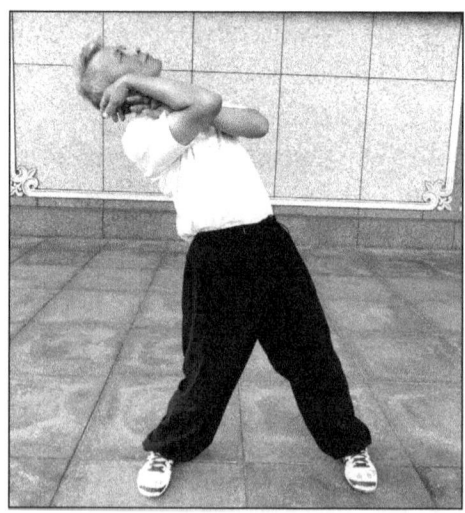

Master Lin Jianhong, a top disciple
of Guo Tingxian, effortlessly transforms
from one animal to another.

References in Chinese

Cheng Jiading (1976). *Laws of health and longevity*. True Perfect publishing. 程家鼎 (1976). [健康長壽法]。真善美出版。

Guo Tingxian (1990). *Hua Tuo's five animal frolics illustrated*. Self-published. 郭廷獻 (1990). [華陀五禽之戲圖解]。台北：自行出版。

Guo Tingxian (1990). *Hua Tuo's five animal frolics instructional video*. The first instructional video of the Five Animal Frolics in Taiwan. Self-published. 華佗五禽戲教學視頻影片。台北：自行出版。

Li Zhangzhi (Feb. 2010). The inheritance and development of Hua Tuo wu qin opera in Taiwan. http://azh57.pixnet.net/blog/post/ 303 91545

Xiong Yiqun (Ed.). (1983). *Martial art collection*. Hong Kong: Joint Publishing. 熊岫雲(1983). [武藝拾]。香港: 聯華出版社出版。

Zhang Jingying (2006). *Calligraphic collection.* Taipei. Self-published. 張鏡影 (2006). [書法文書法文物集]。台北：自行出版。

References - Websites

Chinese Hua Tuo five Animal Frolics Association: http://fatsai.pixnet.net/blog

Daoyin Research Group: http://www.qigong.co.kr/en/index.html

Lin Jianhong: https://www.youtube.com/watch?v=Bh1munRYSEo

Tsou, Jeff: https://jefftsou.pixnet.net/blog

*Note: This chapter was previously published in *Qi: The Journal of Traditional Eastern Health & Fitness* (winter 2018-2019), pp. 38-42; and in the German periodical *Taijiquan & Qigong Journal,* (4-2018), pp. 16-21.

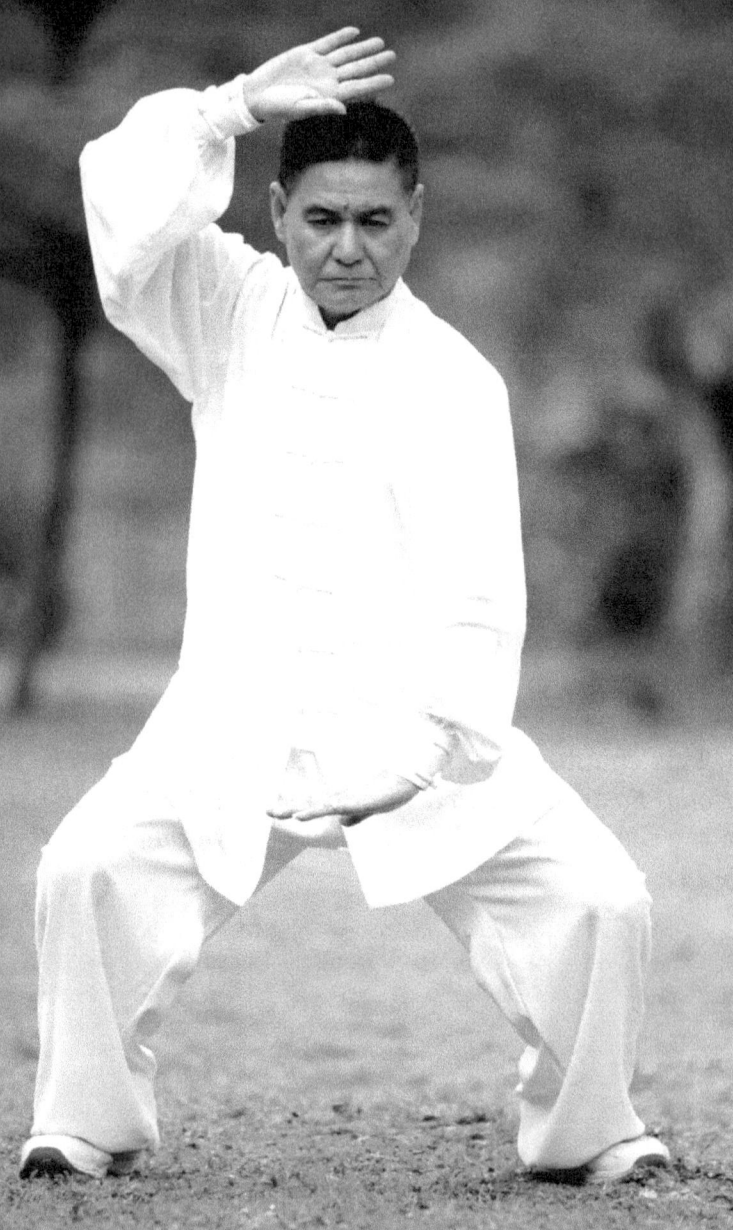

Lin Chaolai

"Standing on the Earth"
posture in Taiji-Qigong practice.

Other Chinese Styles in the Xiong System

Since his childhood, Xiong was open-minded, absorbing all he could regarding martial traditions. He learned from his father, Shaolin masters, taiji masters, and others. In later years, after his move to Taiwan, he continued to study, learn, and share.

One of Xiong's seniors, Master Huang Guozhi, says that it takes a lifetime to learn all the Xiong curriculum. As author of this book, with the handicap of being a foreigner, I certainly have not grasped the totality of the martial regimen. I've seen the practices, but I'm not totally clear on the roots of each.

The styles outside of those taught by Xiong associated with taijiquan are mentioned here only for reference. There are a few additional practices added since his passing. Xiong's senior student Yang Qingyu brought in Chen Panling's 24 Stick (陳泮嶺24式短棍) routine and many in the Xiong lineage practice it today. Even though Master Xiong did not teach the Five Animal Frolics, he encouraged it, and it flourishes among the Xiong lineage.

Other traditional martial art practices from Xiong's teachings:

- Aoguchui   拗股捶
- Baihong Sword   白虹劍
- Bench   板凳
- Chunyang Sword   純陽劍
- Dragon Sword   龍形劍
- Four Gates Hong Boxing   四門洪拳
- Four-Gate Ten Directions Double Sword 四門十路雙劍
- Six-Way Flower Spear   六路花槍
- Spring and Autumn Broadsword   春秋大刀
- Sunlight Palm   曦陽掌等
- Taizu Staff   太祖棍
- Taizu Eighteen Paired Staff   太祖十八對棍

- Wudang Short Staff 武當短棍
- Xiaohong Boxing 小紅拳
- Xiaohua Sword 小花劍
- Xiezhen Secret Sect Fist 寫真秘宗拳
  (Misleading Fist) （迷蹤拳）
- Xingyi Chain Sword 形意連環劍
- Yexing Broadsword 夜行刀
- Yijinjing 易筋經

The Sunlight Palm practices that were passed down from Master Tang Dianqing through Xiong Yanghe are three routines:

- Green-Haired Lion Fist (aka Night Fighting Eight Directions)
  青毛獅拳（又名夜戰八方）

- Stone Fist (aka Seven-Star Plum Blossom Stance)
  石頭拳（又名七星梅花勢）

- Xiliang Palm Fist (aka Xiyang Palm Fist)
  西涼掌拳（又名曦陽掌拳）

Many Xiong Style practitioners have focused solely on the taijiquan curriculum. It is enough for anyone. Nevertheless, the most dedicated remain devoted to preserving the entire syllabus.

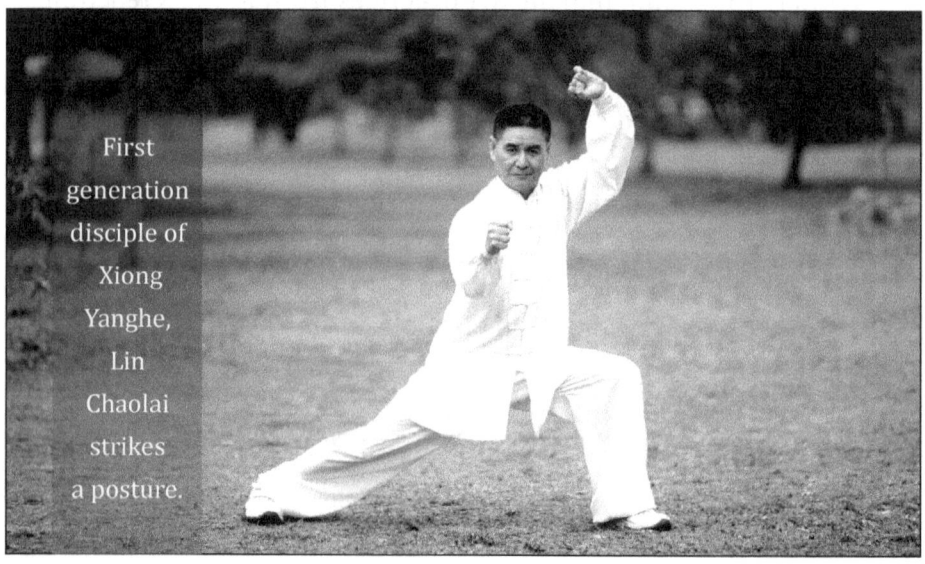

First generation disciple of Xiong Yanghe, Lin Chaolai strikes a posture.

APPENDIX: Partial List of Xiong's First-Generation Disciples

Cao Yanfu	曹衍福	Lu Yuxuan	陸雨軒
Cao Zenghua	曹增華	Lü Zhenzong	呂振宗
Chen Deyang	陳德洋	Ma Tingi	馬廷基
Chen Huang	陳皇	**Meng Shanfu**	孟善夫
Chen Shanyi	陳善一	**Qiu Shuzhou**	裘署舟
Chen Wenxiong	陳文雄	**Rao Shunchen**	饒舜臣
Chen Xiaolan	陳曉蘭	Tang Jianhua	唐建華
Chen Xiaoyin	陳曉寅	**Tao Bingxiang**	陶炳祥
Chen Xinggui	陳興桂	**Wan Xiaoyan**	萬小燕
Chen Xixi	陳錫熙	Wang Huazhong	王華中
Chen Zhenhe	陳珍和	**Wang Jingzhi**	王靜之
Guo Tingxian	郭廷獻	**Wang Juemin**	王覺民
Huang Guozheng	黃國政	Wang Rongbin	王榮賓
Huang Guozhi	黃國治	Wang Tianfu	王天福
Huang Qinglin	黃清麟	Wang Yulin	王玉琳
Huang Zhenghong	黃正宏	**Wei Guang**	魏廣
Huang Shumei	黃淑梅	Wu Songxing	吳淞淬
Jian Tiangong	簡天拱	Wu Xiangqing	吳祥慶
Jin Peiming	金培明	Xie Youxin	謝又新
Liang Dongcai	梁棟材	Xie Chaoqing	謝朝清
Lin Benlie	林本烈	Xiong Wei	熊衛
Li Gongjie	李功杰	Xu Fengyuan	徐逢元
Li Guoguang	李國光	Xu Rongzong	徐榮宗
Li Rixin	李日新	Yang Fuan	楊福安
Lin Chaolai	林朝來	Yang Qingyu	楊清玉
Liu Guqiu	劉古球	Ye Wenkuan	葉文寬
Lin Kun	林坤	Yi Yuehui	易月輝
Lin Lianfu	林連富	Yu Xianquan	俞賢銓
Lin Lianzhi	林連枝	Zhang Lao	張栨
Lin Qingzhi	林清智	**Zhang Nan**	張楠
Lin Shengtian	林勝添	Zhang Rongshu	張榮樹
Lin Songnian	林松年	**Zhang Zhongping**	張仲平
Lin Xianghua	林祥華	**Zhong Dazhen**	鍾大振
Lin Qingxiang	林清祥	Zhu Fu	朱福
Liu Yuan	劉淵	**Zou Xueyuan**	鄒學元
Liu Zhaoji	劉肇基		

APPENDIX: Selected Biographies

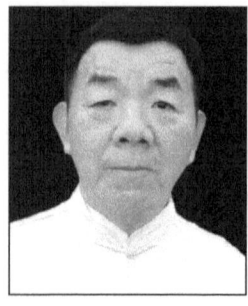

Chen Deyang
陳德洋

In 1960, Chen Deyang (b. 1945), began studying under Xiong Yanghe. Once discussing Buddhism, Xiong told Deyang that he knew much about it, but as he gets older, the understanding of Buddhism changes. It is the same with martial arts. Now that Master Chen is over eighty years old, he is more aware of his teacher's depth of knowledge. Chen Deyang compiled the Yu De Tajji 42 Form. In 1992, he published the book *Yu De Taiji Push Hands and Da Lu*. Chen Deyang has been teaching continously for 66 years.

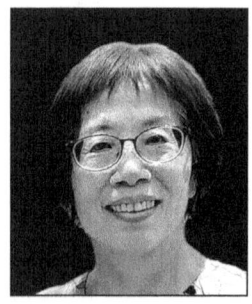

Chen Xiaoyin
陳曉寅

From a young age, Chen Xiaoyin trained in a variety of martial arts styles. Her grandfather knew Xiong Yanghe very well and invited him to live with them in Yonghe city. They were from the same mainland hometown and shared ancestral ties. Miss Chen addressed him as "Second Grandfather." Many senior students visited, offering her many learning opportunities. After graduating from a university, Master Chen entered public service. Following retirement, she taught martial arts at schools, the Sun Yat-sen Memorial Hall, and church.

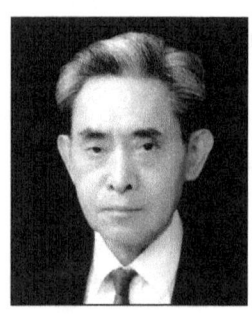

Guo Tingxian
郭廷獻

Guo Tingxian (1925-2002) started to study taijiquan in 1956 with Master Xiong Yanghe and became one of Xiong's top disciples. Before this, he studied in-depth with Zhang Jing-ying who was the 77th generation representative of a health system stemming from the Daoists of Qingcheng Mountain in Sichuan Province. Guo was one of Zhang's five disciples to master the original 125-movement version of the Five Animal Frolics. Guo, in part with the help of Master Xiong, is responsible for spreading Hua Tuo's Five Animal Frolics across the island.

Huang Guozhi started his study with Xiong Yanghe in 1967 when he was twelve years old and became one of the master's top disciples. With over fifty years of experience, Master Huang has been dedicated to promoting and preserving the essence of Xiong's Taijiquan. In addition to regular lessons for his students, he often gives lectures and presentations. He proofread and demonstrated in Xiong's book *Illustrated Guide to Single and Paired Taiji Sword Training*. Master Huang has produced an extensive amount of materials for Xiong's system.

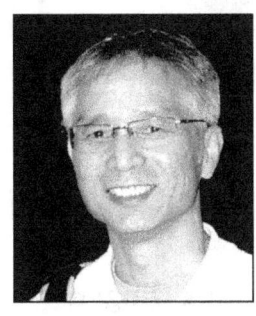

Huang Guozhi
黃國治

Born in 1955, Huang studied with a number of top masters over the decades. His martial art studies is encyclopedic, including Xiong's taiji and Shaolin systems, Five Animal Frolics, and the Buddhist tradition. He was the principal coach of Yilan Taijiquan Association. Huang has produced and extensive reference collection of writings and videos, documenting nearly all the martial styles he has studied over the decades. He tirelessly promotes martial arts and Xiong's legacy.

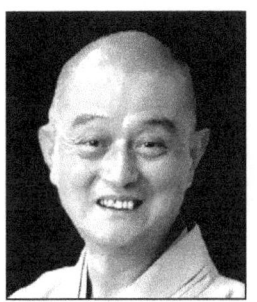

Huang Qinglin
黃清麟

In 1959, Lin Chaolai was six years old and began learning martial arts with Xiong. He formally became his disciple at age thirteen. Lin worked as Former Station Manager at the Taiwan Railways Administration. He also keeps Xiong martial arts on track! He has taken on many responsibilities as Honorary Chairman of the Xiong Family Taji Association of China and served on many other associations, plus acting as an advisor and coach. Retired from his formal employment, Master Lin continues to work full-time promoting Xiong's martial arts.

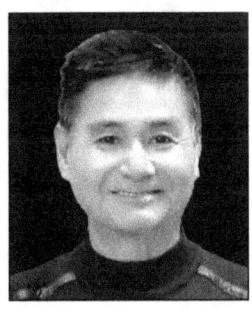

Lin Chaolai
林朝來

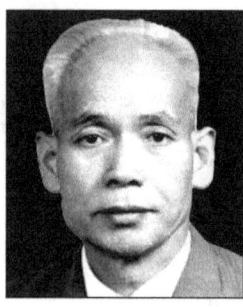

Yang Qingyu

楊清玉

Master Yang in 1986 in Puli city.

Master Yang Qingyu (April 12, 1915–February 6, 2002), was born in Song Village (宋莊), which is located in Sheqi county (社旗县) in the southwestern side of Henan Province. Song Village is about 150 miles from the Shaolin Temple, and 200 miles to Chen Village, the birthplace of taiji. He studied martial arts since his early childhood.

Like Xiong, Master Yang served in the military on the mainland. Following the Chinese Civil War when they settled in Taiwan, Yang became one of Xiong's earliest disciples in Yilan, living in Xiong's home. Yang had severly suffered from rheumatism during the war years and credits Xiong's teaching for his recovery. He praised Xiong for his sympathetic heart, fostered with studies of Buddhist scriptures.

Yang lived and taught in Taipei and after moving to Puli city taught there and other cities in Taiwan. He followed Xiong in the martial ways as wells as the Buddhist teachings.

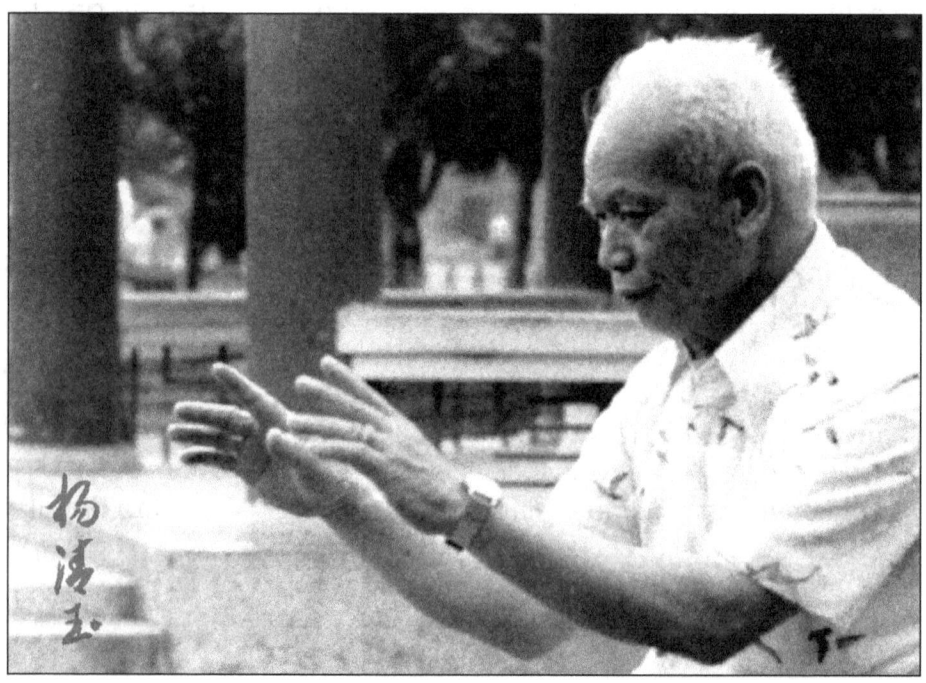

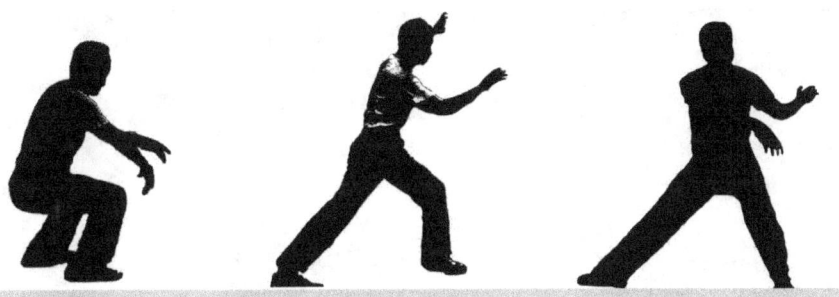

Below left:
Master Yang and the author pose before a statue of General Chennault in New Park in 1976. Lieutenant General Claire Lee Chennault (1893–1958) was an American military aviator who commanded the "Flying Tigers" during World War II in China. Master Yang served in the military during those years of great unrest in China.

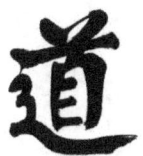

Above: Yang's calligraphy of the character *dao*, the Way.

Below right: Master Yang and the author at the Guanyin (Goddess of Mercy) Buddhist Temple, in Puli, central Taiwan. Photo date May 21,1989.

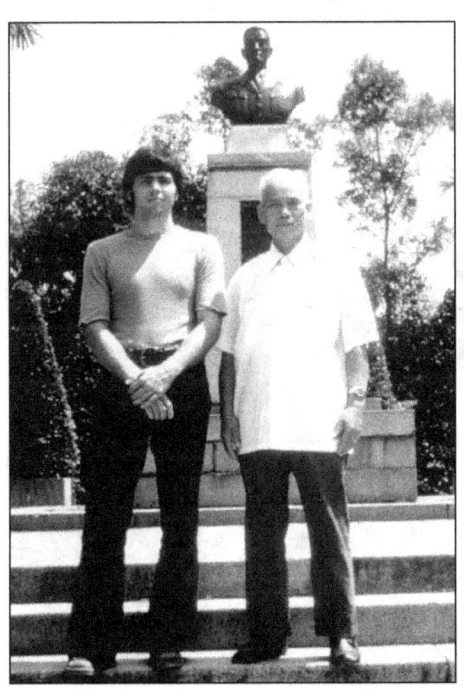

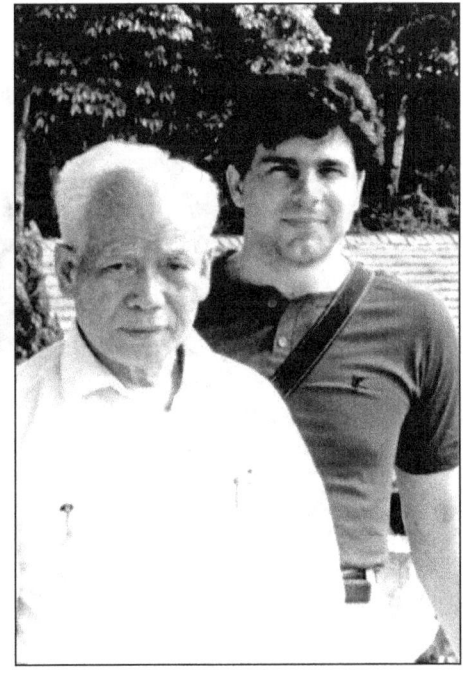

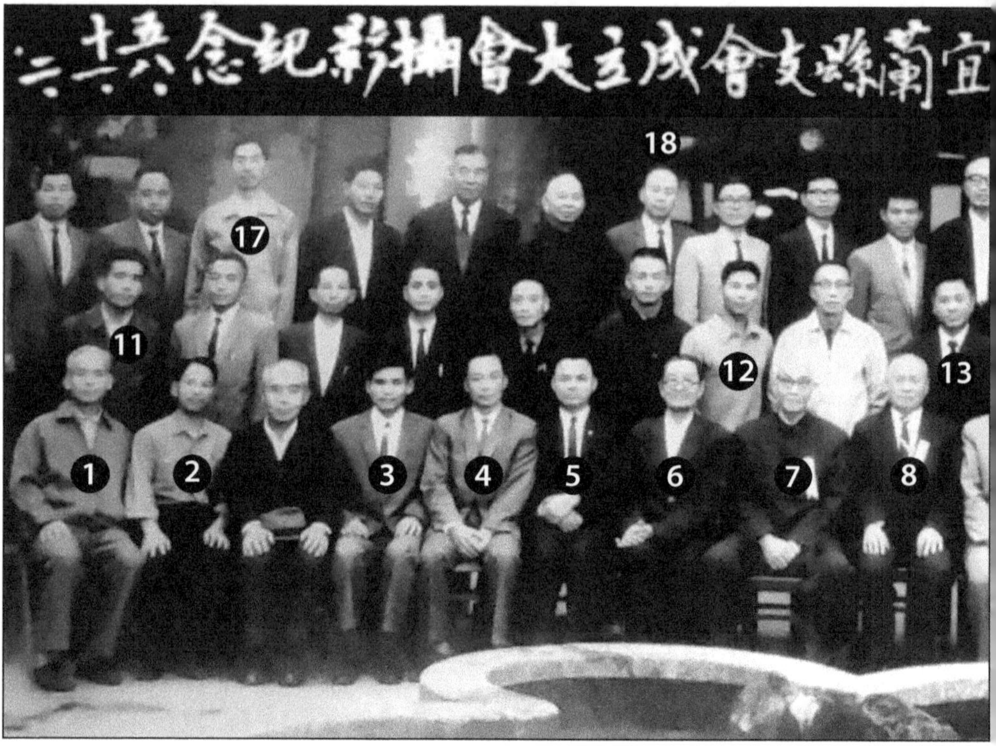

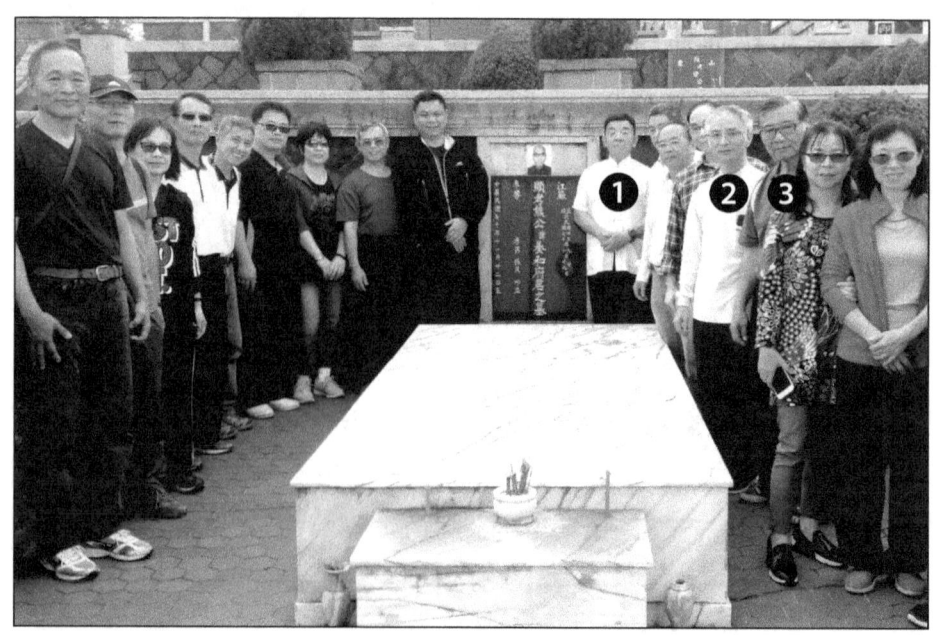

1) 楊清玉 2) 俞賢銓 3) 林連富 4) 張大文 5) 鍾去非 6) 劉古球 7) 熊養和
8) 韓振聲 9) 王覺民 10) 陳國民 11) 張柟 12) 林清智 13) 饒舜臣 14) 呂振宗
15) 簡天拱 16) 陳皇17) 林本烈 18) 陳錫熙 19) 林連枝 20) 林朝來 21) 鄧志誠

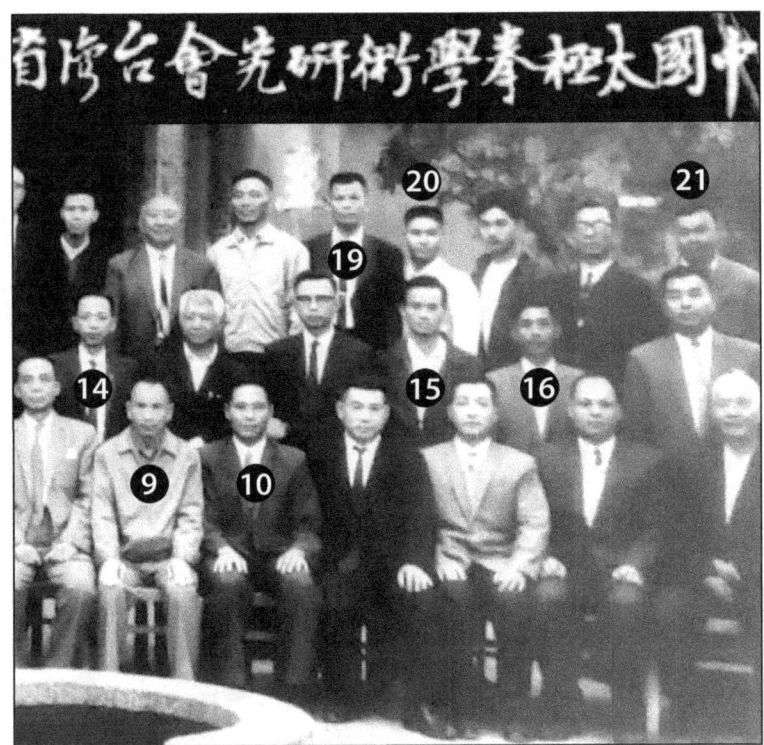

1) Yang Qingyu
2) Yu Xianquan
3) Lin Lianfu
4) Zhang Dawen
5) Zhong Qufei
6) Liu Guqiu
7) Xiong Yanghe
8) Han Zhensheng
9) Wang Juemin
10) Chen Guomin
11) Zhang Nan
12) Lin Qingzhi
13) Rao Shunchen
14) Lu Zhenzong
15) Jian Tiangong
16) Chen Huang
17) Lin Benlie
18) Chen Xixi
19) Lin Lianzhi
20) Lin Chaolai
21) Deng Zhicheng

Yilan County Branch of the Chinese Taiji Academic Research Association.
Photograph from the founding meeting, 11/2/1969.

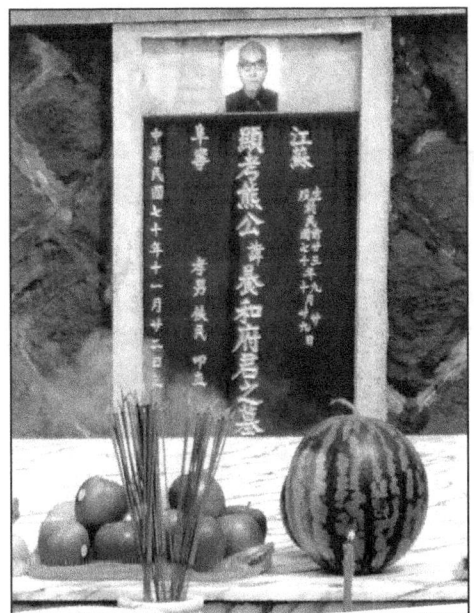

Previous page, bottom:
(1) Chen Deyang,
(2) Huang Guozhi and
(3) Lin Qingzhi led their students to pay their respects at the grave of their master Xiong Yanghe. All bring offerings and perform the formal "Three Kneels and Nine Kowtows."

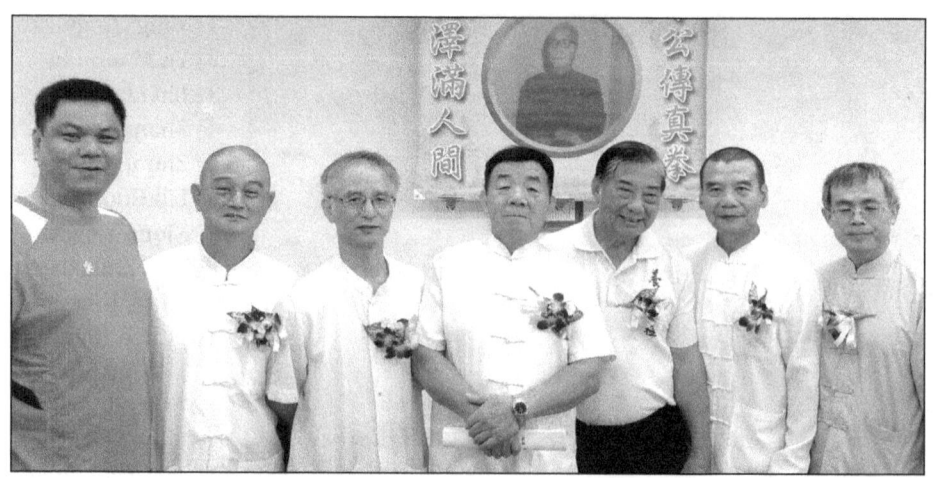

L to R: Xiong Yanghe's great grandson Xiong Naiqi; Xiong's seniors: Huang Qinglin, Huang Guozhi, Chen Deyang, Lin Qingzhi, and Li Guoguang; and Xiao Futang.

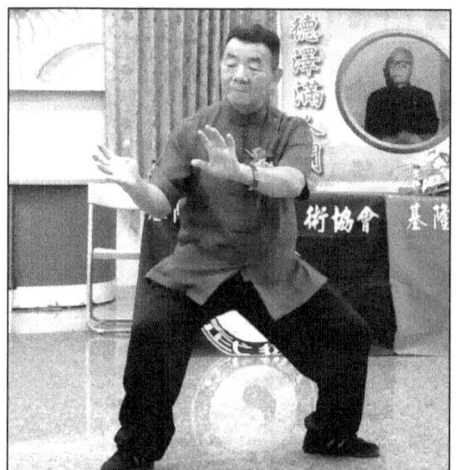 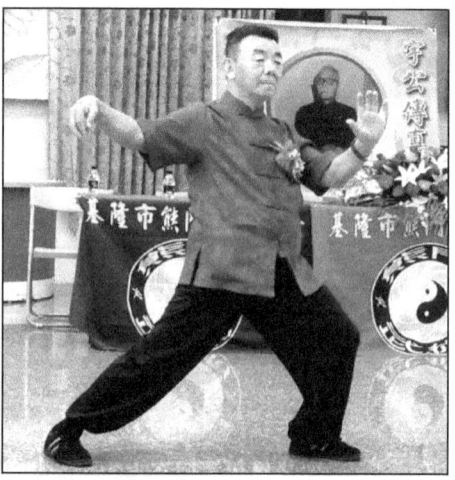

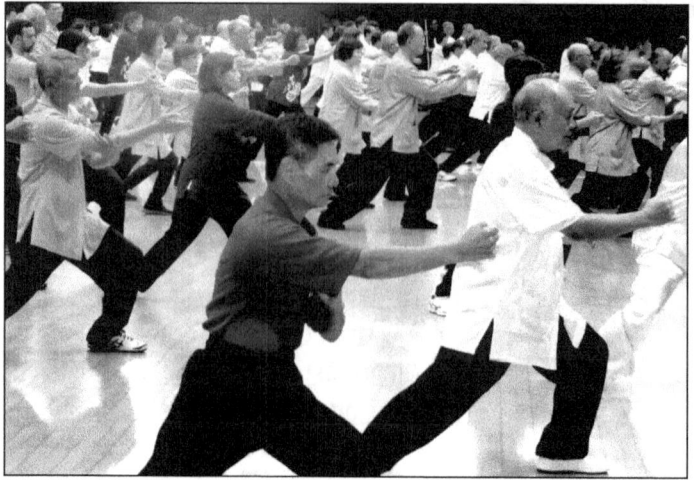

Above: Chen Deyang. Left: Lin Chaolai and other seniors leading a group during the 130th anniversary celebration gathering for Grandmaster Xiong.

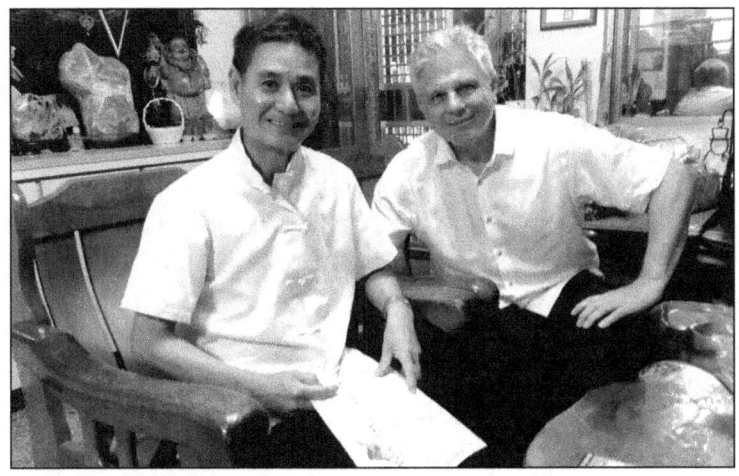

Lin Chaolai generously sharing documents about the Xiong history and practice with the author during a visit to his home.

Below: Huang Qinglin and the author practicing sanshou.
Lin Chaolai open-hand form and Huang Guozhi with taiji sword.

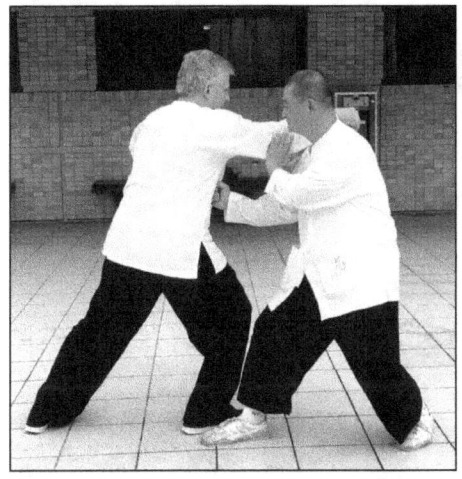
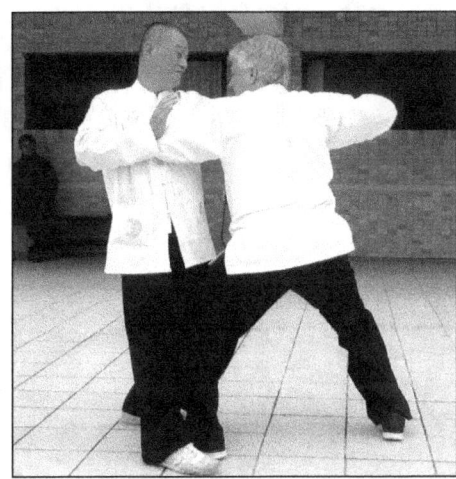
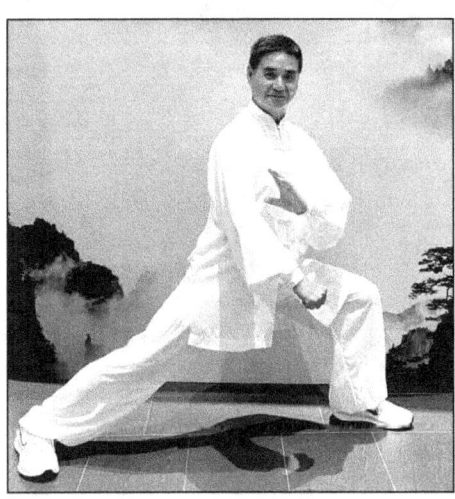
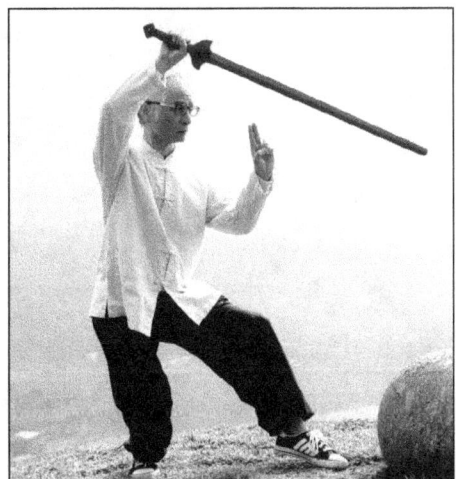

105

130th ANNIVERSARY CELEBRATION for Grandmaster Xiong Yanghe

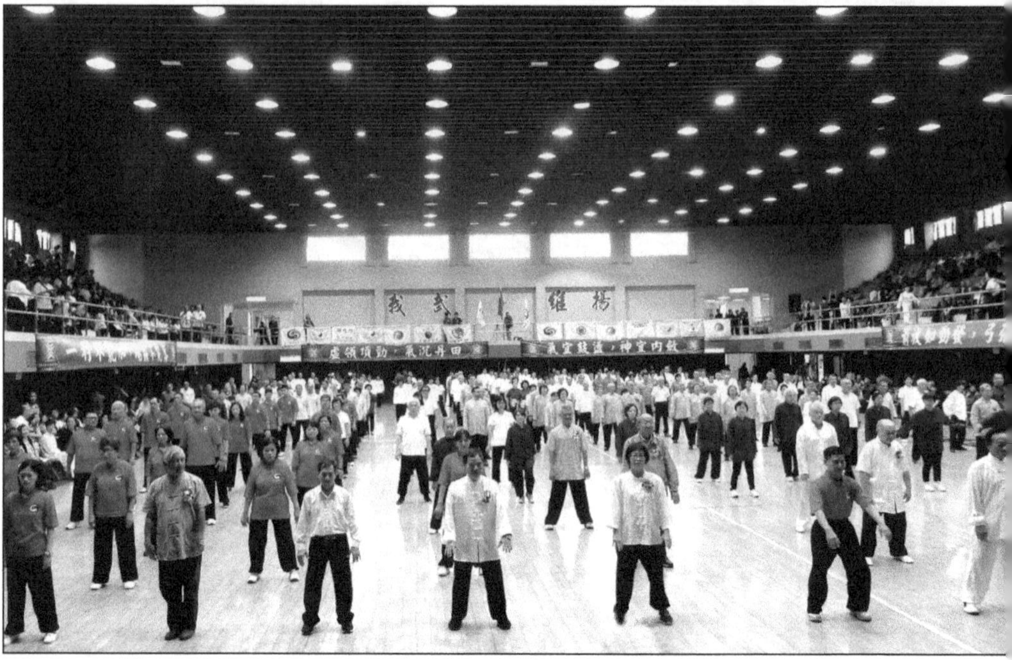

Below, at a banquet gathering, left to right: Zhong Minghai (鍾明海), the author, Lin Chaolai (林朝來), Lin Changxiang (林昌湘) and Huang Junwei (黃俊維).

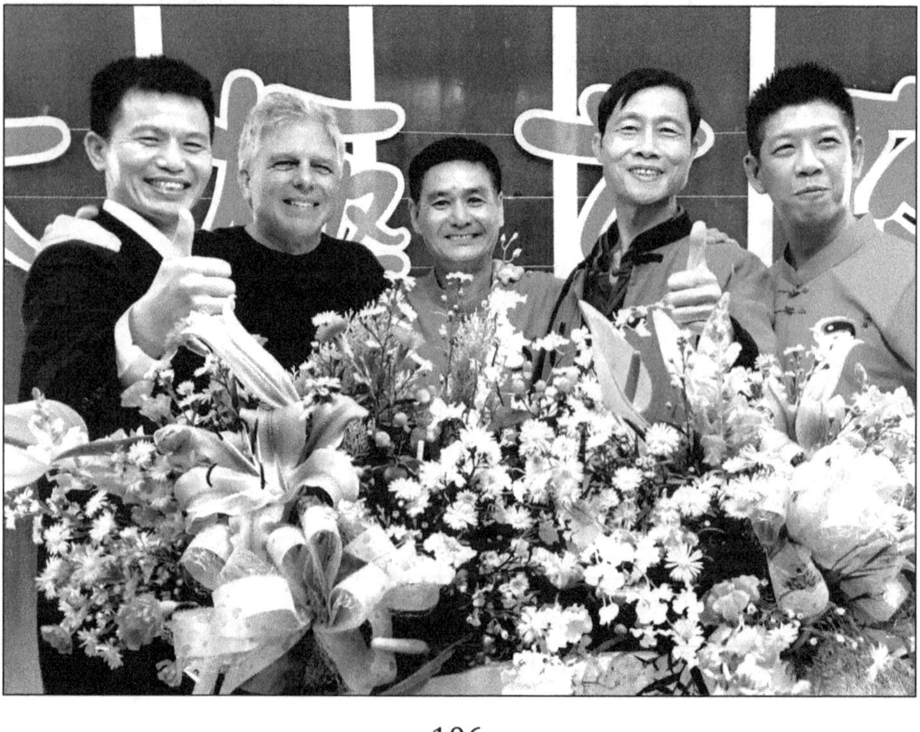

Held in Yilan, Taiwan, November 4, 2017

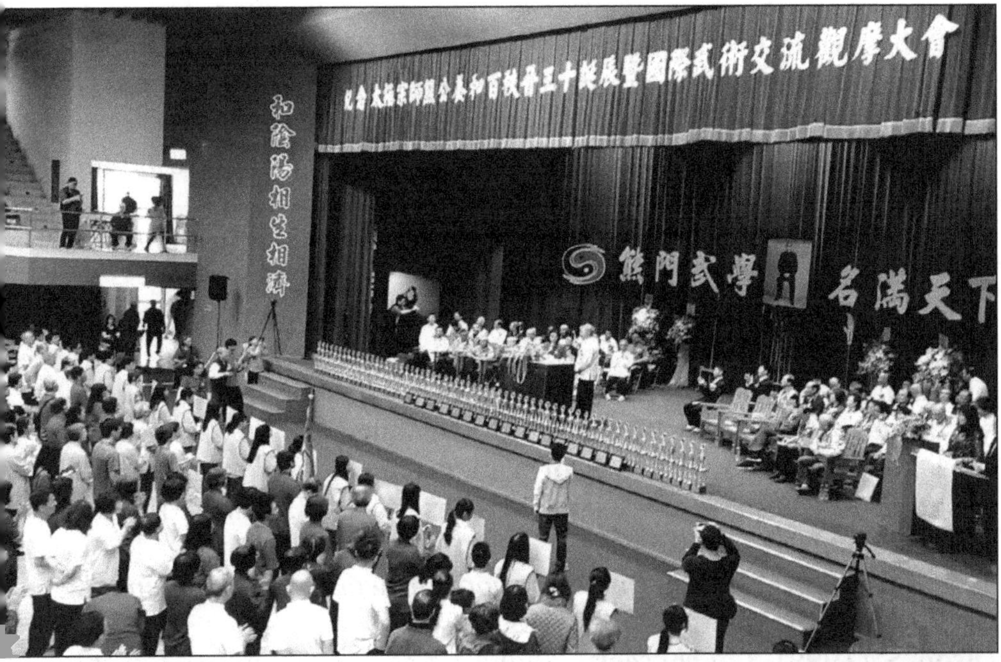

Above and right: the author at the podium for at the 130th anniversary celebration.

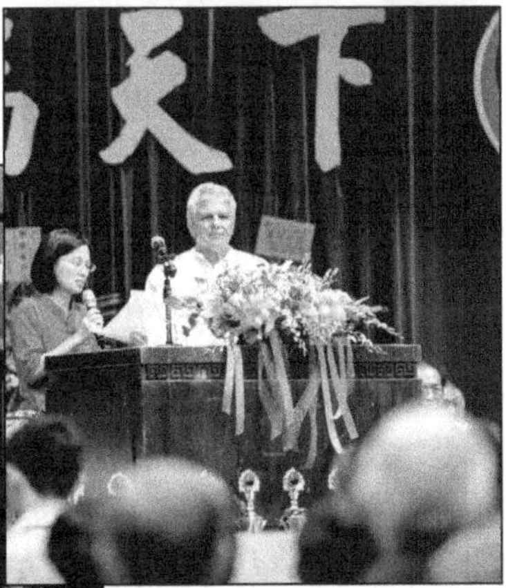

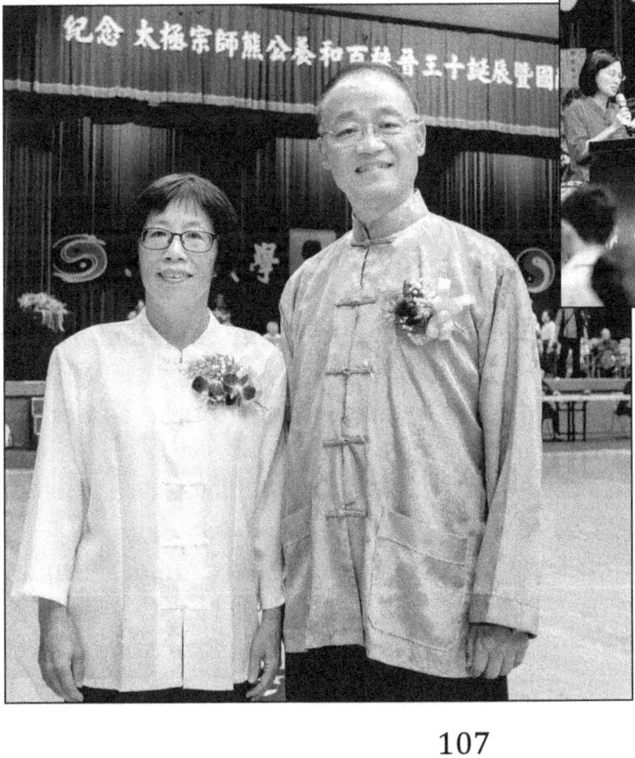

Left: Master Chen Xiaoyin (陳曉寅) with one of her protégés, Pan Taichun (潘台春), who teaches at the Harmony Tai Chi Center in Concord, Massachusetts.

Selected Reference Materials - English

Chen Qingzeng (n.d.). *Explanation of traditional five animal exercises.* Published by Chen Qingzeng.

DeMarco, M. (1992). The origin and evolution of taijiquan. *Journal of Asian Martial Arts,* 1(1): 8-25.

Gallagher, P. (2007). *Drawing silk: Masters' secrets for successful tai chi practice.* Charleston, SC: BookSurge.

Guo Tingxian (1980). *Illustrated guide to Hua Tuo's Five Animal Exercises.* Published by Guo Tingxian.

Hayward, R. (2000). *T'ai-chi ch'uan: Lessons with master T.T. Liang.* St. Paul, MN: Shu-Kuang Press.

Kurland, H. (May 1998). "Hsiung Yang-Ho's san shou form." *T'ai chi Ch'uan and Wellness Newsletter.* Downloaded July 16, 2009.

Kurland, H. (2003). "History of a rare t'ai-chi form: San shou." http://www.self-growth.com/articles/Kurland3.html. Downloaded July 16, 2009.

Olson, S. (1999). *T'ai chi thirteen sword: A sword master's manual.* Burbank, CA: Multi-Media Books.

Olson, S. (1999). *T'ai chi sensing-hands: A complete guide to t'ai chi t'ui-shou training from original Yang Family records.* Burbank, CA: Multi-Media Books.

Olson, S. (1992). *The teachings of master T.T. Liang: Imagination becomes reality, the complete guide to the 150-posture solo form.* St. Paul, MN: Dragon Door Publications.

Russell, J. (2004). *The tai chi two-person dance: Tai chi with a partner.* Berkeley, CA: North Atlantic Books.

Selected Reference Materials – Chinese

Anonymous (2017). *Master Xiong's 130th birthday commemorative special edition.* (n.p.). Also DVD Set was published.

Anonymous (1987). *Master Xiong's 100th birthday commemorative special edition.* (n.p.).

Anonymous (1984). *National arts master Xiong Yanghe commemorative collection.* (n.p.).

Cheng Jiading (1976). *Laws of health and longevity.* True Perfect publishing. 程家鼎 (1976). [健康長壽法]。真善美出版。

Guo Tingxian (1990). *Hua Tuo's five animal frolics illustrated.* Self-published. 郭廷獻 (1990). [華陀五禽之戲圖解]。台北：自行出版。

Guo Tingxian (1990). *Hua Tuo's five animal frolics instructional video.* The first instructional video of the Five Animal Frolics in Taiwan.

Self-published. 華佗五禽戲教學視頻影片。台北：自行出版。

Li Zhangzhi (Feb. 2010). The inheritance and development of Hua Tuo wu qin opera in Taiwan. http://azh57.pixnet.net/blog/post/ 303 91545

Lin, Caolai (2007). *Yang family old frame Xiong style taijiquan*. DVD. Yilan, Taiwan: Chin-yu Martial Art Study Association.

Yang, Qingyu (1976). Xiong style taijiquan long form, push-hands, and sword form. Private film collection.

Yang, Qingyu (1988). *Yang Qingyu autobiography*. Self-published.

Yang, Qingyu (n.d.). *A brief biography of Xiong Yanghe*. Self-published.

Xiong, Yanghe (1962). *Xiong Yanghe autobiography*. Self-published.

Xiong, Yanghe (1963). *The taijiquan explained*. Taipei: Taiwan China Book Printing House.

Xiong, Yanghe (1971). *Taiji swordsmanship illustrated*. Yilan, Taiwan: Lu Feng Printing and Publishing House.

Xiong Yanghe (1973). *Illustrated explanation of taiji sword technique*. Published by Xiong Taisheng.

Xiong, Yanghe (1975). *Taijiquan explained*. 3rd edition. Taipei: Huge Distribution Planning Company.

Xiong Yanghe (1977). *Illustrated guide to single and paired taiji sword exercises*. Published by Xiong Taisheng.

Xiong Yiqun (Ed.). (1983). *Martial art collection*. Hong Kong: Joint Publishing. 熊岫雲(1983). [武藝拾]。香港: 聯華出版社出版。

Website Sources

DeMarco, Michael. https://www.wingedliontaichi.com

Huang, Guozhi (黃國治). https://xn--sssq1u1mfc0co3j.app/ https://熊氏太極拳.app

Huang, Qing (黃清麟) . https://g0919902131.wixsite.com/happy-martialarts

Pan, Taichun (潘台春). https://taichipan.wixsite.com/taichifor-health

Xiong Yanghe Photographs

As part of its goal to maintain cultural records, Taiwan's National Digital Archives Program (see www.ndap.org.tw) has digital photographs of Xiong Yanghe in the collection which can be viewed in thumbnail and large format (view at http:/ digitalarchives.tw).

INDEX

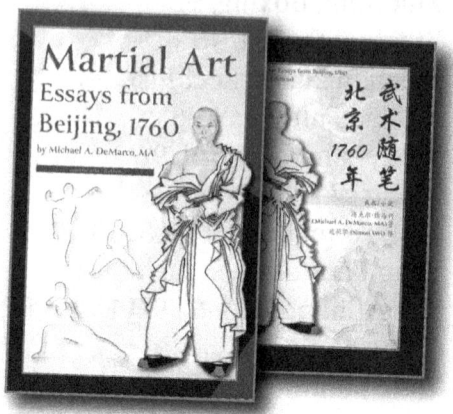

Martial Art Essays from Beijing, 1760

English & Chinese Editions

"DeMarco leads us on a journey into the world of sacred wisdom that we all sought when we first joined the martial arts. This text rivals the importance of classics like *The Art of War* and *Book of Five Rings*..."
➡️**Kevin Secours,** founder of Integrated Fighting Systems, Canada

"... important and thrilling to read."
➡️**Stephan Berwick,** founder, True Taiji; martial arts culturalist and advocate

"In this book, the power and ingenuity of Chinese fighting arts flow open before our eyes in precise, engaging text...."
➡️**Manuel Adrogué, LLD,** Taekwon-Do seventh dan, Argentina

"Absolutely riveting."
➡️**Nicklaus Suino,** founder Japanese Martial Arts Center, Ann Arbor, Michigan

"DeMarco reveals the physical, technical, psychological, and philosophical elements of the internal arts..."
➡️**David Gaffney,** founder Chenjiagou Taijiquan GB, England

"This work not only lays out the principles of practice in a clear and concise manner, it does so in an entertaining format that includes history, intrigue, and first-person instruction from the masters of the past."
➡️**Tim Cartmell,** founder of Shen Wu Martial Arts; head, BJJ/MA coach at Ace Jiu Jitsu Academy

FORMAT: 5.25" x 8" paperback, 144 pages, 27 illustrations

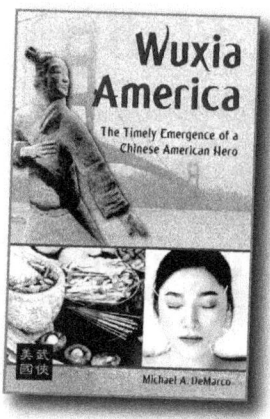

Wuxia America
The Timely Emergence of a Chinese American Hero

"*Wuxia America* is an exciting ride intertwining culture, history, medicine, martial arts, and mystery. DeMarco's novella draws on the *wuxia* theme of using martial arts for justice through Dr. Lou's reluctant heroism, while also delving into the cultural connections between China and America, and the contributions Chinese Americans have made to society. — Richly engaging."
➡**David Hazard, Ph.D.** Stanford University
Department of East Asian Languages and Cultures

"Internationally renowned author and martial arts savant Michael DeMarco brings his considerable prose talents to the wonderful novella form with a tale powered by his expertise, his world travels and a river that powers much of great fiction: the quest. And in *Wuxia America*, that quest helps us align our lives in a direction more meaningful and spiritually fulfilling as human beings."
➡**James Grady**, author of *Six Days of the Condor* and *This Train*

"DeMarco's new book *Wuxia America* amazed me greatly while reading through the well written pages. The book includes touching stories of the early Chinese in America and an underlying theme of the principles and spirit about the *wuxia* — martial heros. It is both interesting and educational reading. I recommend the book highly."
➡**Edwin Pak-wah Leung, Ph.D.**
Full Professor Emeritus of Asian Studies, Seton Hall University

FORMAT: 5" x 8" paperback, 152 pages, 27 illustrations

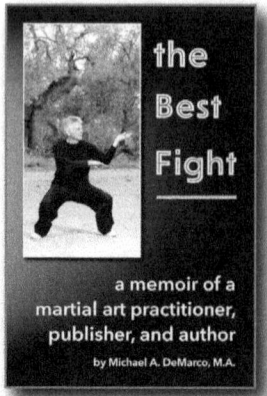

The Best Fight

a memoir of a
martial art practitioner,
publisher, and author

A needle may draw a thread through printed pages to bind a book. In this little memoir, I feel like a needle that drew a common thread though a segment of martial art history. This book details three interrelated activities: (1) martial art studies, (2) involvement as founder of Via Media Publishing, producing a quarterly journal and books, and (3) teaching martial arts.

Publishers, writers, researchers and serious martial art practitioners will benefit with the detailed overview of Via Media and its publications. Via Media produced the **Journal of Asian Martial Arts**, known for its high academic and aesthetic standards. Its contents reflect the history of two decades and provides rich information for practitioners and scholars, making **The Best Fight** a valuable reference work.

In addition to reading, the primary way to learn a martial art is through instruction. In reading about my studies and teaching experience, readers can relate to their own involvement in martial arts. What is important here is the portrayal of my instructors, their teaching methods, and reasons for being involved in martial arts. Their accounts should offer insights and inspiration for others who study and practice any martial art.

Books by Michael DeMarco
are available directly from:
www.viamediapublishing.com
Amazon and other online stores.

FORMAT 6"x9" paperback, 140 pages, 65 illustrations

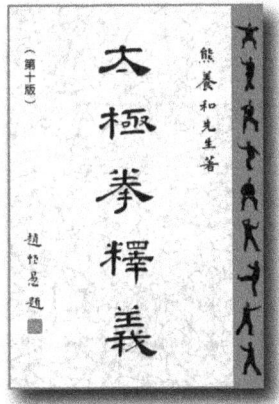

太極拳釋義 (第十版)
Taijiquan: An Interpretation
(10th Edition)

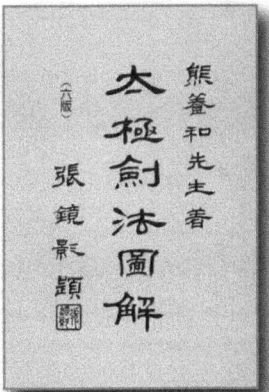

太極劍法圖解 (第六版)
Taiji Straight Sword Methods Illustrated
(Sixth Edition)

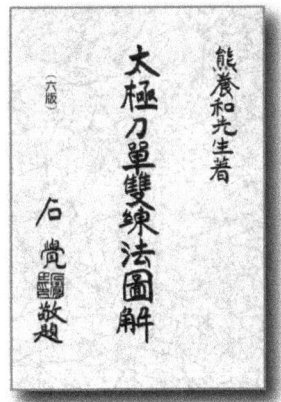

太極刀單雙練法圖解 (第六版)
Illustrated Solo and Paired Taiji Broadsword Practices (Sixth Edition)

To order

If you want more information or to order any of the titles, please contact Mr. Xiong Naiqi at:
Email: naichi.hsiung@gmail.com

有需要的朋友請洽 熊哥老師:
Email: naichi.hsiung@gmail.com
https://feebee.com.tw • https://biggo.com.tw

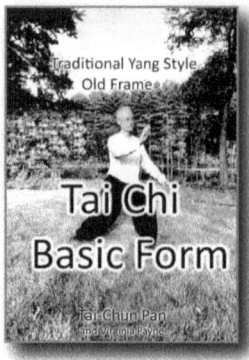

Traditional Yang Style Old Frame Tai Chi Basic Form

by Taichun Pan (潘台春) and Virginia Payne

This book explains the traditional Yang Style Taiji passed down by grandmaster Xiong Yanghe. Mr. Tai-chun Pan has been practicing taijiquan since 1968 and teaching in the Greater Boston area since 1980. In Taiwan, he studied directly under Masters Chen Xiaoyin and David Cheng.

FORMAT: 7"x10"paperback, 135 pages, illustrated
See details on Amazon.com

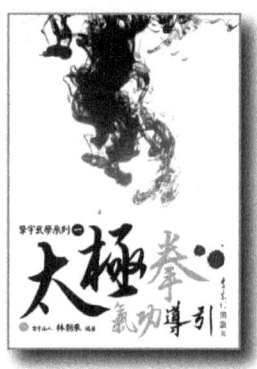

太極拳氣功導引 (書籍和DVD) 林朝來作者
Taijiquan Qigong Daoyin (book and DVD) by Lin Chaolai

FORMAT: 7.5" x 10.25" paperback, 128 pages, illustrated. Queries for this title and his other available books and DVDs, contact Master Lin Chaoli by email: chaolai@kimo.com

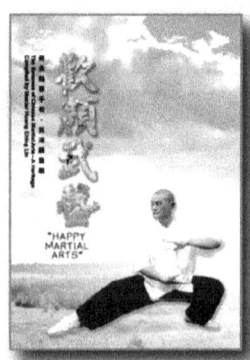

歡顏武藝 黃清麟 作者
Happy Face Martial Arts by Huang Qinglin

FORMAT:
8.25"x11.5" paperback, 151 pages, illustrated

Free download link:
https://g0919902131.wixsite.com/happymartialarts/blank-1

Notes